Sexually Transmitted Diseases

EDITED BY

RICHARD H. BEIGI MD, MSc

Associate Professor of Reproductive Sciences
Divisions of Reproductive Infectious Diseases and Obstetric Specialties
Department of Obstetrics, Gynecology and Reproductive Sciences
Magee-Womens Hospital of the University of Pittsburgh Medical Center
Pittsburgh, PA, USA

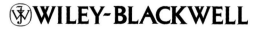

A John Wiley & Sons, Ltd., Publication

This edition first published 2012, © 2012 by John Wiley & Sons, Ltd.

Wiley-Blackwell is an imprint of John Wiley & Sons, formed by the merger of Wiley's global Scientific, Technical and Medical business with Blackwell Publishing.

Registered office: John Wiley & Sons, Ltd, The Atrium, Southern Gate, Chichester, West Sussex, PO19 8SQ, UK

Editorial offices: 9600 Garsington Road, Oxford, OX4 2DQ, UK
The Atrium, Southern Gate, Chichester, West Sussex, PO19 8SQ, UK
111 River Street, Hoboken, NJ 07030-5774, USA

For details of our global editorial offices, for customer services and for information about how to apply for permission to reuse the copyright material in this book please see our website at www.wiley.com/wiley-blackwell

Library of Congress Cataloging-in-Publication Data
Sexually transmitted diseases / edited by Richard H. Beigi.
    p. ; cm. – (Gynecology in practice)
  Includes bibliographical references and index.
  ISBN 978-0-470-65835-2 (pbk. : alk. paper)
  I. Beigi, Richard H.   II. Series: Gynecology in practice.
  [DNLM: 1. Sexually Transmitted Diseases–diagnosis. 2. Sexually Transmitted Diseases–therapy. WC 140]

  616.95′1–dc23

                                                                    2012002551

A catalogue record for this book is available from the British Library.

Wiley also publishes its books in a variety of electronic formats. Some content that appears in print may not be available in electronic books.

Set in 8.75/11.75 pt Utopia by Thomson Digital, Noida, India
Printed and bound in Malaysia by Vivar Printing Sdn Bhd
1 2012

Contents

List of Contributors

Richard H. Beigi, MD, MSc
Department of Obstetrics, Gynecology and
Reproductive Sciences,
Magee-Womens Hospital of the University
of Pittsburgh Medical Center
Pittsburgh, PA 15213, USA

Carolyn Gardella, MD, MPH
Department of Ob/Gyn
Division of Women's Health
University of Washington
Box 356460
Seattle, Washington 98195-6460, USA

Suzanne M. Garland
Department of Microbiology and Infectious
Diseases, The Royal Women's Hospital,
Parkville, Victoria 3052, Australia
Department of Obstetrics and Gynaecology,
University of Melbourne, Parkville, Victoria,
Australia
Murdoch Children's Research Institute,
Parkville, Victoria, Australia

Alice Goepfert, MD
Professor
Department of Obstetrics and Gynecology
Division of Maternal-Fetal Medicine
619 19th Street South, 176F 10270N
Birmingham, AL 35249-7333, USA

Ravi Gunatilake
Duke University Hospital
Durham, North Carolina, USA

R. Phillip Heine
Duke University Hospital
Durham, North Carolina, USA

Lisa M. Hollier, MD, MPH
Professor, Maternal-Fetal Medicine
Department of Obstetrics, Gynecology and
Reproductive Sciences
University of Texas Houston Medical School
LBJ General Hospital
5656 Kelley Street
Houston, TX 77026, USA

Katherine M. Holman, MD
Instructor
Department of Medicine
Division of Infectious Diseases
University of Alabama at Birmingham
1900 University Blvd, THT 229
Birmingham, AL 35294, USA

Oluwatosin Jaiyeoba, MD
Department of Obstetrics and Gynecology
Medical University of South Carolina
Charleston, South Carolina, USA

Noor Niyar N. Ladhani, MD MPH FRCSC
Fellow, Maternal Fetal Medicine
University of Toronto
Toronto, Canada
2108-1055 Bay St
Toronto, Ontario M5S 3A3, Canada

Eduardo Lara-Torre, MD, FACOG
Associate Professor of Obstetrics and
Gynecology
OBGYN Residency Program Director
Virginia Tech Carilion School of Medicine
1906 Belleview Ave
Roanoke, VA 24014, USA

Tracy L. Lemonovich, MD
Instructor of Medicine, Division of Infectious
Disease and HIV Medicine
University Hospitals Case Medical Center,
Case Western Reserve University
11100 Euclid Ave, Cleveland, OH 44106, USA

Silvia T. Linares, MD
Assistant Professor
Department of Obstetrics, Gynecology &
Reproductive Sciences
University of Texas Houston Medical
School
LBJ General Hospital
5656 Kelley Street
Houston, TX 77026, USA

Jeanne M. Marrazzo, MD, MPH
Professor of Medicine, Division of Allergy &
Infectious Diseases
Harborview Medical Center, Division of
Infectious Diseases
325 Ninth Avenue, Mailbox #359932
Seattle, WA 98104
And
Medical Director, Seattle STD/HIV
Prevention Training Center
University of Washington, Seattle, WA, USA

Michelle H. Moniz, MD
Department of Obstetrics, Gynecology and
Reproductive Sciences,
Magee-Womens Hospital of the University
of Pittsburgh Medical Center

Amber Naresh, MD, MPH
Department of Obstetrics, Gynecology &
Reproductive Sciences
Division of Reproductive Infectious Diseases
University of Pittsburgh
300 Halket Street
Pittsburgh, PA 15213, USA

Robert A. Salata, MD
Professor of Medicine, Division of
Infectious Disease and HIV Medicine
University Hospitals Case Medical Center,
Case Western Reserve University
11100 Euclid Ave, Cleveland,
OH 44106, USA

Ashlee Smith, DO
Gynecologic Oncology Fellow
300 Halket Street
Magee-Womens Hospital
Division of Gynecologic Oncology
Pittsburgh, PA 15213, USA

Jack D. Sobel, MD
Division of Infectious Diseases
Harper University Hospital
3990 John R
Detroit, MI 48201, USA

David E. Soper, MD
Medical University of South Carolina
Department of Obstetrics and Gynecology
96 Jonathan Lucas Street, Suite 634
P.O.Box 250619, Charleston, SC 2942, USA

Glenn Updike, MD, MMM
Assistant Professor
Department of Obstetrics, Gynecology, and
Reproductive Sciences
University of Pittsburgh
Suite 0892
Magee-Womens Hospital
300 Halket Street
Pittsburgh, PA 15232, USA

Mark H. Yudin, MD MSc FRCSC
Associate Professor, University of Toronto,
Department of Obstetrics and Gynecology
Attending Physician, St. Michael's Hospital,
Department of Obstetrics and Gynecology
Toronto, Canada
30 Bond Street
Toronto, Ontario M5B 1W8, Canada

Kristin K. Zorn, MD
Assistant Professor, Department of Obstetrics,
Gynecology and Reproductive Sciences
300 Halket Street
Magee-Womens Hospital
Division of Gynecologic Oncology
Pittsburgh, PA 15213, USA

Series Foreword

In recent decades, massive advances in medical science and technology have caused an explosion of information available to the practitioner. In the modern information age, it is not unusual for physicians to have a computer in their offices with the capability of accessing medical databases and literature searches. On the other hand, however, there is always a need for concise, readable, and highly practicable written resources. The purpose of this series is to fulfill this need in the field of gynecology.

The *Gynecology in Practice* series aims to present practical clinical guidance on effective patient care for the busy gynecologist. The goal of each volume is to provide an evidence-based approach for specific gynecologic problems. "Evidence at a glance" features in the text provide summaries of key trials or landmark papers that guide practice, and a selected bibliography at the end of each chapter provides a springboard for deeper reading. Even with a practical approach, it is important to review the crucial basic science necessary for effective diagnosis and management. This is reinforced by "Science revisited" boxes that remind readers of crucial anatomic, physiologic or pharmacologic principles for practice.

Each volume is edited by outstanding international experts who have brought together truly gifted clinicians to address many relevant clinical questions in their chapters. The first volumes in the series are on *Chronic Pelvic Pain*, one of the most challenging problems in gynecology, *Disorders of Menstruation*, *Infertility*, and *Contraception*. These will be followed by volumes on *Sexually Transmitted Diseases*, *Menopause*, *Urinary Incontinence*, *Endoscopic Surgeries*, and *Fibroids*, to name a few. I would like to express my gratitude to all the editors and authors, who, despite their other responsibilities, have contributed their time, effort, and expertise to this series.

Finally, I greatly appreciate the support of the staff at Wiley-Blackwell for their outstanding editorial competence. My special thanks go to Martin Sugden, PhD; without his vision and perseverance, this series would not have come to life. My sincere hope is that this novel and exciting series will serve women and their physicians well, and will be part of the diagnostic and therapeutic armamentarium of practicing gynecologists.

Aydin Arici, MD
Professor
Department of Obstetrics, Gynecology, and
Reproductive Sciences
Yale University School of Medicine
New Haven, USA

Preface

Sexually transmitted diseases (STDs) have been recognized for centuries, are the subject of many ancient writings, and have likely been present for at least as long as humans, given the necessity of human reproduction. Early descriptions of syphilis, gonorrhea, herpes simplex virus, and other STDs (and their associated clinical syndromes) have been found in both medical and nonmedical documents. On a global scale, STDs remain one of the most prevalent infectious diseases among the human race. Despite numerous technological advances in the past century, including the introduction of effective antimicrobial agents, STDs persist, and even thrive in varied locales.

There are numerous obstacles internationally to the successful control of STDs, including, in many instances, social, financial, and political underpinnings complicating control efforts. The health threats posed by many STDs also frequently extend to unborn fetuses and/or neonates, increasing their global importance. Because of the substantial prevalence of many of these clinical entities, as well as the significant toll on health and associated societal costs, clinicians caring for girls and women of all ages should have a thorough working knowledge of STD recognition, diagnosis, and management.

For the typical women's health provider, STDs and their associated morbidities represent a sizable portion of the daily efforts directed at improving and maintaining health, in addition to treating acute ailments. Also, many clinical efforts focus on STDs as a part of the larger goal of promoting disease prevention among women. In addition to the well-known STDs, the infectious vulvovaginitis syndromes are a major cause of discomfort, remain one of the main reasons women seek care and use antimicrobial agents, and are thus discussed thoroughly. Given significant overlap in clinical presentation, many noninfectious conditions of the female genital tract are also commonly seen by busy women's health providers and are occasionally misdiagnosed as STDs and/or infectious vulvovaginitis. This is also true for the relatively rare, but clinically apparent, vulvovaginal cancers. The awareness of these noninfectious clinical entities has increased in recent years, and burgeoning research has demonstrated the relatively high frequency of many of these conditions. Thus, special attention is given in this text to some of these more common entities.

Taken together, these conditions require a thorough understanding and disciplined approach to the evaluation and management in order to optimize women's health globally. Importantly, human immunodeficiency virus (HIV), while a sexually transmitted pathogen, is not discussed directly in this text, primarily because its scope and breadth warrants an entire text unto itself.

It is my sincere hope that this text provides a thorough yet user-friendly guide to the common STDs, vaginitides, and the gynecologic noninfectious syndromes that are frequently encountered in clinical practice. I also hope and believe that the combination of excellent contributors, along with the unique chapter selections, will serve as an invaluable resource for busy women's health providers across the world.

Richard H. Beigi, MD, MSc

Standard Clinical Evaluation

Richard H. Beigi

Department of Obstetrics, Gynecology and Reproductive Sciences, Magee-Women's Hospital of the University of Pittsburgh Medical Center, Pittsburgh, PA, USA

Introduction

The clinical evaluation of women presenting with genital tract complaints requires a standard approach that leads to an objective, reproducible evaluation. This is a critical point to understand given the diverse conditions that are being evaluated. These diverse conditions, however, often have very closely overlapping clinical presentations, requiring the standard approach to maximize diagnostic accuracy and optimize outcomes. In general, the evaluation of women with lower genital tract complaints without physical examination and/or laboratory testing has been demonstrated to be suboptimal. Self-diagnosis has also been demonstrated to be inaccurate, and is generally discouraged. The syndromic management of women, based on subjective presentation alone, has been used in developing countries (and still is in certain settings) where a health infrastructure is lacking. However, thorough and careful history-taking, physical examination, and selected laboratory methods can significantly improve objectivity and, whenever possible, are strongly recommended in developed nations with an existent healthcare infrastructure. A recommended and reproducible approach to all women with lower genital tract complaints is described below.

Clinical evaluation

A thorough understanding of the vulvar, vaginal, and internal female genital tract anatomy is the key first step in assessingvulvovaginal complaints among women. As noted in Figure 1.1, the vulva is bound by the genitocrural folds laterally, the anus posteriorly, and the upper mons pubis superiorly. Importantly, hair follicles (coarse) are present on the inferior, lateral, and superior tissues of the vulva, but are lacking from the inner labia majora, labia minora, and the vaginal vestibule. The vaginal vestibule is separated from the inner labia minora by an artificial anatomic line, called the Hart line. This is an important landmark because it separates the nonmucous-secreting outer skin from the inner, mucous-secreting moist tissues of the vaginal vestibule and the hymenal ring. The vaginal vestibule is where the Bartholin and minor vestibular glands are located and produce lubricating fluids, where the vaginal orifice begins, and where the urethra opens at its meatus. Delineating and appreciating the exact anatomical location of physical findings is very important in deciphering the underlying etiology as well as administering effective treatment of sexually transmitted diseases (STDs) and the associated vulvovaginal syndromes/conditions.

Sexually Transmitted Diseases, First Edition. Edited by Richard H. Beigi.
© 2012 John Wiley & Sons, Ltd. Published 2012 by John Wiley & Sons, Ltd.

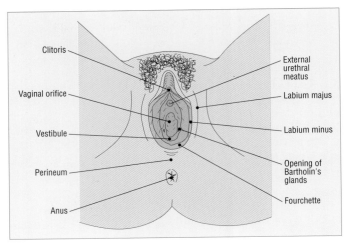

Figure 1.1. Female external genitalia. (Reproduced from Rogstad KE, et al., *ABC of Sexually Transmitted Infections,* 6th edn. Blackwell Publishing: Oxford, 2011, with permission.)

The standard position for most gynecological examinations is the dorsal lithotomy (on back, with knees flexed, thighs flexed and apart, feet resting in stirrups). This positioning (Figure 1.1) allows in most scenarios the best physiologic view of the female anatomy and optimizes specimen collection for most laboratory analyses. Occasionally, due to anatomic restrictions, lack of mobility, or other factors, different positioning may be necessary or undertaken. This may be especially true for young women or girls who have never had pelvic examinations performed or are reticent for such an examination (covered more extensively in Chapter 2).

It is likewise essential for practitioners caring for women to have a thorough understanding of the internal female genital tract anatomy (Figure 1.2). This cross-section demonstrates the relationship of the vagina, cervix, uterus, and adnexae to each other as well as the relationship to the two other important organ systems in the pelvis – the gastrointestinal tract (large bowel) and the urinary system (urethra and bladder). Distinguishing signs and/or symptoms attributable to the genital

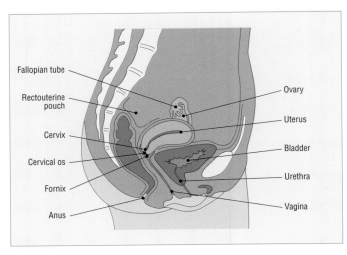

Figure 1.2. Female internal genitalia. (Reproduced from Rogstad KE, et al., *ABC of Sexually Transmitted Infections,* 6th edn. Blackwell Publishing: Oxford, 2011, with permission.)

tract versus the other adjacent organ systems is often challenging but occasionally very important to successful management.

With this basic understanding of the female anatomy, history-taking becomes the next key step (as in nearly all clinical evaluations). Focusing on specific symptomatology, exact timing of the onset of symptoms and length of time, alleviating and exacerbating factors, recent therapies (including self-chosen and nonprescription remedies) and presence/absence of partner(s) symptoms will help to narrow the differential diagnoses. The Centers for Disease Control and Prevention (CDC) has recommended an approach to sexual history-taking (5 Ps), which is covered more extensively in Chapter 17 (Prevention of Sexually Transmitted Diseases). This approach is strongly recommended to assist providers' ability to obtain key information in these evaluations that will lead to the correct diagnosis and management, thus improving clinical outcomes. Use of nonjudgmental, open-ended questions is suggested when eliciting a sexual history as this approach is more likely to produce meaningful and accurate information about sexual practices and risk factors.

After taking a thorough history and with a thorough understanding of the anatomy, all evaluations begin with an inspection of the vulvar area. Close attention to all elements of the external genital anatomy, the presence of any lesions, appearance and color of the skin, labia majora and minora, as well as any atypical findings is required. Obvious large lesions or other major findings should be noted and captured in a drawing for future reference. More subtle findings such as fissuring, labial agglutination, or small ulcers should also be sought, as they often give direct insight into the etiology of symptoms. Lymph nodes in the inguinal region should be routinely palpated for enlargement and/or tenderness (or rarely, fluctuance). For some of the vaginitides (i.e. vaginal candidiasis) and especially the noninfectious and/or dermatologic conditions, vulvovaginalinspection is often a high-yield component of the examination. After a thorough examination of the vulvar tissues (specific attention to color, tissue appearance, lesions, scaling, etc.), the vaginal introitus should be inspected for color changes, the presence of lesions, and vaginal tissue rugosity (as a sign of endogenous estrogen stimulation).

Subsequent to the thorough inspection of the external anatomy and vaginal introitus, anappropriately sized speculum should be placed into the vaginal vault, and the vaginal tissues and cervix inspected. Again, attention to tissue color, texture, presence of discharge, anatomic origin of the discharge (vaginal vs. cervical os), and other signs should be noted on every patient. Origin of discharge is a key point, as cervical discharge has a vastly different etiology, evaluation, and management compared to discharge emanating from the vaginal tissues. Evaluation of discharge microscopically is also a very important component of nearly all genital tract evaluations (when considering infectious conditions) and can often yield highly valuable information. The specifics of these techniques will be discussed in ensuing chapters. Close attention to the cervical appearance is also a key to this part of the examination. Once this is performed (and any appropriate specimens obtained for testing), the speculum is removed.

Internal bimanual pelvic examination is then carried out in the usual fashion using two fingers in the posterior vagina to palpate and move the cervix, while placing the other hand on the lower abdomen to simultaneously palpate the internal genital organs. This component of the examination is done with specific attention to the findings of pelvic tenderness on motion of the cervix (i.e. cervical motion tenderness) and any adnexal and/or uterine findings. This too is an important part of the examination that can often give vital information about upper genital tract infection that requires specific (often prolonged) therapy. Rectovaginal examination is also an often used method to help to discern further the nature of any findings on pelvic examination, as well as specific findings in the anorectal canal itself, and should be used liberally.

Conclusion

Use of this standard and reproducible approach on every patient will improve the ability of the provider to objectively determine the cause of the symptomatology. This in turn will improve the management and patient outcomes from these often physically and psychologically debilitating conditions.

Specific Considerations for Pediatric and Adolescent Patients

Eduardo Lara-Torre

Department of Obstetrics and Gynecology, Virginia Tech Carilion School of Medicine, Roanoke, VA, USA

Introduction

The management of sexually transmitted infections (STIs) in children and adolescents requires the practitioner to apply a different approach from the one used for adult women.

To understand the screening and treatment algorithms, one must understand some basic epidemiology and behaviors that differentiate these patients from their counterparts. It is also important to understand the indications, techniques, and alternative methods of screening utilized with this population, especially because these patients may be hesitant to be screened and examined in the traditional way. When dealing with children and adolescents, understanding local law and state statutes regarding the confidentiality of their reproductive healthcare is also important as it dictates the type of services they can receive without parental notification and also determines the rules and regulations for reporting. This is not only noted in the presence of certain infections such as chlamydia, but more importantly among those patients who might have been victims of sexual abuse.

In general, children are screened and treated for STIs related to involuntary intercourse or genital contact. Examples of these inappropriate contacts may include sexual abuse with penetration or simply the placement of male genitals in contact with the child's vulva. The management of children with STIs requires a multidisciplinary approach and should include collaboration between the governmental agencies (such as child protective services), laboratory, and clinicians. Some infections acquired after the neonatal period are consistent with sexual abuse (i.e. gonorrhea), while other diseases such as HPV may not be. A full understanding of the management of victims of sexual abuse is important for those caring for this population and is beyond the spectrum of this chapter.

Adolescents, on the contrary, are more commonly screened and treated for acquired infections due to consensual sex. The approach to each of these scenarios is different, and the evaluation and management for each patient and conditions will be presented in separate sections.

The physical examination

Prepubertal girls

The initial step in the examination of children is to obtain the cooperation of the child. While explaining the examination to the patient, allow her to have some say in the process (e.g. give the child a choice of examination gown to wear).

Sexually Transmitted Diseases, First Edition. Edited by Richard H. Beigi.

© 2012 John Wiley & Sons, Ltd. Published 2012 by John Wiley & Sons, Ltd.

Starting with an overall assessment of the child before initiating the genitalia examination is recommended as it will provide an opportunity for the patient to become comfortable with the examiner and proceed with the genital examination.

In order to be able to visualize the genitalia of children, positioning plays a key component to the success of the examination. Multiple positions have been described to allow adequate visualization, and, in some situations, more than one position may be required to complete an adequate genital examination. The frog-leg is the most commonly used position in the younger patient, allowing her to have a direct view of the examiner and herself (Figure 2.1). The knee–chest position is adjunctively helpful in some cases in visualizing the lower and upper vagina with the use of an otoscope or other low-power magnification. This position may be especially helpful in those patients for whom a vaginal discharge may be a complaint (Figure 2.2). As the child grows older, the use of stirrups and the lithotomy position may provide the best visualization of the area. Having the mother hold her daughter on her lap may also be of assistance. In certain instances, even the most experienced examiner will be unable to complete the examination because the child will not fully cooperate. In these patients, the emergent nature of the complaint and the clinical consequence of the pathology must be considered. A multivisit examination or an examination under anesthesia may be warranted.

The use of gentle traction with lateral and downward pulling may improve visualization while maintaining the integrity of the normal prepubertal genitalia (Figures 2.3 and 2.4). The examiner must be careful not to cause any trauma or pain in the area, as it will promptly make the patient uncomfortable and possibly lead to a premature termination of the examination. In the prepubertal female, the unestrogenized nature of the hymenal tissue makes it sensitive to touch and easily torn.

Although the evaluation of the internal pelvic organs may not be easy, the use of a recto-abdominal examination may assist in the palpation of the internal organs as well as possible pelvic masses. Proper nomenclature of the female genitalia should be used when reporting a pediatric genital examination to prevent confusion between examiners. Components of such an examination include assessment of pubertal development (Tanner stage), visualization and measurement of the clitoris, and description of the labia majora and minora including any discoloration, pigmentation, or lesion. The appearance of the urethra, meatus, and hymen (including type or shape, estrogen status, and abnormalities) should be detailed. Estrogenization at puberty thickens the hymen, which

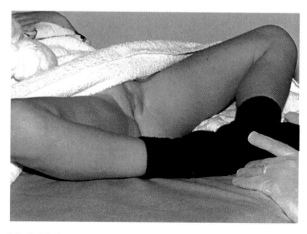

Figure 2.1. A 5-year-old child demonstrating the supine "frog-leg" position. (Reproduced from McCann JJ, Kerns DL. *The Anatomy of Child and Adolescent Sexual Abuse: A CD-ROM Atlas/Reference*, Intercort, Inc.: St. Louis, MO, 1999 with permission.)

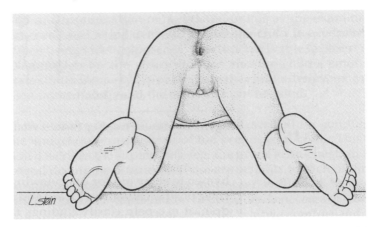

Figure 2.2. Technique for examination of female genitalia in prone knee–chest position. (Reproduced from Finkel MA, Giardino AP (eds.). *Medical Examination of Child Sexual Abuse: A Practical Guide*, 2nd edn. Sage Publications: Thousand Oaks, CA, 2002; pp. 46–64, with permission.)

becomes pale pink and is often more redundant in its configuration, but in the prepubertal patient the hymen is thin, red, and unestrogenized. If the cervix is visualized in the knee–chest position, it is important to document its appearance.

Using special techniques to obtain specimens

The hymenal opening is small in this age group, and traditional cotton swabs create discomfort. When vaginal specimens for culture must be collected, moistened small Dacron swabs (male urethral size) may be used as they are thin and easy to insert without touching the hymen. While making the collection of the sample less traumatic, the accuracy of the test does not change. Another helpful method is a catheter-within-a-catheter technique in which a 4-inch intravenous catheter is inserted into the proximal end of a No. 12 red rubber bladder catheter. This is then connected to a fluid-filled syringe passed carefully into the vagina. The fluid is then injected and aspirated multiple times to allow a good

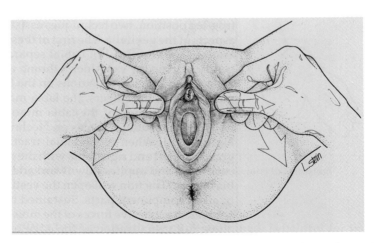

Figure 2.3. Labial traction technique for examination of female genitalia in the supine frog-leg position. (Reproduced from Finkel MA, Giardino AP (eds.). *Medical Examination of Child Sexual Abuse: A Practical Guide*, 2nd edn. Sage Publications: Thousand Oaks, CA, 2002; pp. 46–64, with permission.)

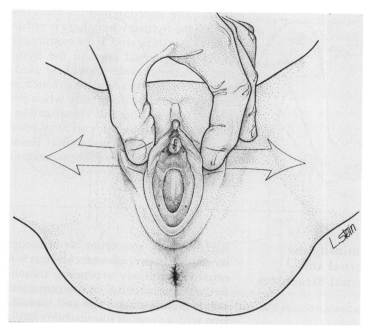

Figure 2.4. Labial separation technique for examination of female genitalia in the supine frog-leg position. (Reproduced from Finkel MA, Giardino AP (eds.). *Medical Examination of Child Sexual Abuse: A Practical Guide*, 2nd edn. Sage Publications: Thousand Oaks, CA, 2002; pp. 46–64, with permission.)

mixture of secretions. These specimens may be sent for culture as needed without affecting the sensitivity or specificity of the tests (Figure 2.5).

As some children age, they may be able to tolerate more office procedures without the need for sedation. In this case, a pediatric feeding tube connected to a 20-mL syringe filled with warm water or saline may be used to irrigate the contents of the vagina and collect the secretions for culture or wash out small pieces of foreign body material such as toilet paper. This can make the need for specula unnecessary in these prepubertal patients who have a small hymenal aperture that would be injured with the insertion of a speculum.

★ TIPS & TRICKS

- When collecting specimens in children, moisten your swabs.
- Do not touch the hymen or you may lose the patient as she may not tolerate the remainder of your examination.
- If using water for vaginal rinse make sure it is warm.

When documenting the findings of the examination and anatomical variations one should merely described the findings and not make

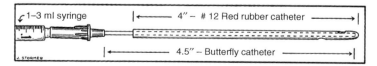

Figure 2.5. Assembled catheter-within-a-catheter aspirator, as used to obtain samples of vaginal secretions from prepubertal patients. (Reproduced from Pokorny SF, Stormer J: Atraumatic removal of secretions from the prepubertal vagina. *Am J Obstet Gynecol* 1987; **156:** 581–582, © 1987 Mosby with permission.)

diagnosis in the examination portion of the documentation. This process of documenting prevents the assumption of abuse and limits the record to a description of the findings.

Vaginal discharge in prepubertal girls

One of the most common complaints in girls seeking gynecological evaluation at this age is vaginal discharge. Vulvovaginitis in children has very different etiology than in adolescents/adults. The main difference in these patients is the etiology of the discharge. While most of the discharge in reproductive-age women is secondary to a specific cause (i.e. yeast, bacterial vaginosis, etc.), the most common etiology in children is a "nonspecific vaginitis."

Local irritation and immaturity of the mucosa probably play a role in the development of the discharge. Its appearance is commonly clear to yellow and may or may not present with itching and odor. Many patients do not even complain about it, but is noticed by the parent in their underwear, leading to concern. Detergents, toilet paper, moisture, perfume, even tight clothing have all been associated with the discharge and discomfort. Hygienic measures in general resolve the problem and no further intervention is necessary. Interventions for the management of nonspecific vaginitis can be found at www.naspag.org.

Bacterial colonization is also a common agent in this condition. Unlike the adult, yeast is rarely encountered in these patients and is present only in those immunosuppressed or on chronic treatment with steroids or antibiotics. Fecal (*E. coli*) or upper respiratory flora (Group A streptococci or *Hemophilus. influenzae*) are the most common bacteria encountered in culture. When hygienic maneuvers fail, a trial of antibiotic treatment for 10 days using such products as amoxicillin or trimetropin/sulfamethoxazole is indicated. If a bloody discharge is present, suspicion for shigella should be considered and an appropriate culture taken. Failure to resolve the symptoms should alert the practitioner to other causes such as foreign body or perhaps organisms associated with sexual abuse.

Adolescent

The adolescent patient may present a challenge for the examining practitioner. The patient's self-consciousness about her own body and the extreme variation in psychosocial and sexual development at this age may make the examination even more difficult to perform. As teenagers develop at varying rates, careful interviewing and counseling should precede an examination. The use of educational videos that explain the examination process and the common reasons why it is done may improve the provider–patient relationship. Delaying the genital examination, even if sexually active, may prevent the patient from having reservations about her examiner. These preferences should be taken into account to make the experience as minimally traumatizing as possible. The examination can be delayed until an indication is present, such as a vaginal discharge or abnormal bleeding or the need for cervical cancer screening has been reached (age 21). Performing an external examination may be undertaken annually as part of the patient's preventive visit. Developing rapport with the teens during their first few visits will allow them to feel ready for this part of their physical examination but the timing will vary from patient to patient.

With adolescents, if possible, it is important to meet initially with the teen and her parents/guardian together to explain the concept of confidentiality and privacy. After the initial history form is completed with parent and teen together, take the sensitive/confidential part of the history with the teen without the presence of the parent (e.g. alcohol, drug and substance use, dating, and sexual history). Remember, when screening, begin with less sensitive issues like safety (e.g. seat belt use) before psychological and sexuality issues.

Before completing the initial gynecologic examination, take time to explain the general process. Patients may choose to delay their pelvic examination when asymptomatic, but the proper examination equipment for this age group should be available if needed. The use of tampons prior to the examination in the presence of menses may facilitate the use of a speculum, as the patient may be more comfortable with vaginal manipulation. A Huffman speculum (1/2 inch wide × 4 inches long) or a Pederson speculum (7/8 inch wide × 4 inches long) may be used with those who are sexually active. Care should be undertaken to utilize the appropriate size speculum for the patients. Teenagers often receive their first-time examination in an urgent or emergency room care setting, where the availability of these smaller instruments may be limited and larger instruments are used, such as the Graves speculum. This practice can lead to an increase in trauma to the patient and apprehension for the pelvic examination, leading adolescents to be reluctant to seek reproductive services for fear of another examination.

Use of the "extinction of stimuli" approach may be of benefit in those undergoing their first pelvic examination. Using a finger to apply pressure to the perineal area, away from the introitus or thigh, will lessen or diffuse the sensation from the examiner's finger at the vaginal opening. Once a finger has been placed in this area, the insertion of a speculum may be easier and the cervix and vagina can be visualized adequately. Once access to the cervix is obtained, cultures may be collected if indicated.

All adolescents should be reassured that the examination, while uncomfortable, is not painful, and will not alter their anatomy. This will reassure those who may believe that the examination will alter their "virginity." After the examination, it is helpful to meet again with the family and patient to explain the findings of the examination and to plan further management. If confidentiality is a concern with the sexually active teenager, first discuss findings with the patient alone while in the examination room.

Sexual assault in children and adolescents

Among patients in whom sexual abuse is suspected, screening and management should include an initial examination at the time of the assault followed by a repeat evaluation 2 weeks after the event. This would allow for those organisms not detected in the original examination to accumulate enough concentration to be detected. Inspection of the genitalia and other possible areas of genital contact from a perpetrator should be undertaken. Suspicious areas of discharge, odor, or lesions must be assessed and samples collected for laboratory analysis. Only specific tests should be used in children as most of the evidence collected will be used in court to pursue criminal charges, and requires little room for misinterpretation.

Initial and 2-week post-event screening should include testing for *Neisseria gonorrheae* and *Chlamydia trachomatis* from the anus, vagina, and pharynx. The use of culture-specific media for the organism is preferred and the use of DNA amplified techniques is discouraged. The Centers for Disease Control and Prevention in 2010 described utilizing Nucleic Acid Amplification Tests (NAATs) as an alternative to *C. trachomatis* culture, with specimens obtained from urine instead of the vagina, potentially minimizing trauma during the examination. At this point, there is insufficient data to support NAAT for *N. gonorrheae* for this indication, and discussion with the local authorities before collection of the specimens is advised to minimize retesting. Collecting a vaginal swab for *Trichomonas vaginalis* culture and bacterial vaginosis is also advisable. During the initial evaluation, collection of serum for human immunodeficiency (HIV), syphilis, and Hepatitis B virus baseline status is recommended. This test can be later compared to samples at 6 weeks, 3 months, and 6 months to detect seroconversion and form an association with the assault.

⚠ CAUTION!

When collecting specimens for cases of sexual abuse, be sure to use organism-specific cultures and not the kits used in adults. This will minimize problems during a trial that could arise because of a lack of gold standard status for nonculture methods. If you are collecting evidence, ensure that the forensic nurses are available to maintain the integrity of the evidence collected.

Prophylaxis after assault is different in children than in any other population. The immature nature of the female anatomy appears to be protective for ascending infection. When making the decision to use prophylactic medications to prevent the acquisition of disease, especially for HIV, it should be in consultation with the parents after an accurate assessment of the risk of acquisition from the perpetrator has been made, and after obtaining consultation from a clinician specializing in infectious diseases in children. Routine prophylaxis without first obtaining verification via accepted testing modalities is not recommended for any disease.

In contrast, prophylaxis for an adolescent who has been the victim of sexual abuse is recommended. Protection against trichomonas, chlamydia, and gonorrhea infections, as well as pregnancy preventions, is advised. Post-exposure use on anti-HIV medications may be indicated but still requires the expertise of those specializing in infectious diseases.

☆ TIPS & TRICKS

When using prophylaxis to prevent STIs in adolescents after sexual abuse use:

- Azithromacin 1 g oral single dose or doxycycline 100 mg oral BID for 7 days for chlamydia.
- Ceftriaxone 250 mg IM or cefixime 400 mg oral single dose for gonorrhea.
- Metronidazole 2 g oral single dose for trichomonas.
- Levonorgestrel 1.5 mg oral single dose for emergency contraception.

Adolescent screening guidelines

In order to optimize care, understanding the indications and testing methodology utilized to screen for STIs in adolescents is important. Having an understanding as to the incidence of certain diseases in this age group justifies the need for asymptomatic screening. High risk-taking behaviors also tend to occur in this age group; in fact adolescents age 15–19 have the highest rates of chlamydia and gonorrhea infections. Adolescents frequently lack access to healthcare. Serial monogamy (i.e. having one partner at the time, but changing partners frequently) and lack of consistent use of barrier methods, increases their overall risk. There also appears to be an increase in susceptibility of the genital tract to acquire some sexually transmitted infections, possibly because of an inherent biological immaturity of these tissues.

An additional complicating issue is that adolescents often seek strict confidentiality when seeing providers for STI management. Although the 50 states and D.C. allow for confidential testing without the need to notify parents of the care or results of the testing, true confidential services are difficult to provide. While the visit information can be kept strictly confidential, the billing resulting from the provider's fee and laboratory testing likely will reach their care givers and/or parents. These invoices will interfere with the confidentiality of the service provided. Some agencies that provide free services to teenagers may be better equipped to handle true confidential services, as no billing is generated for those visits.

Examples of such facilities may include certain planned parenthood clinics and health department STI clinics. These locations may be an ideal option for those teenagers truly concerned about parental discovery. Screening recommendations are listed in Table 2.1.

Table 2.1. CDC screening recommendations for adolescents

- Annual routine screening for *C. trachomatis* on all sexually active patients 25 years old or younger.
- Annual routine screening for *N. gonorrheae* on all sexually active females at risk for STDs at any age.
- HIV risk should be discussed and assessed with all patients at least annually and testing encouraged on all sexually active teens and those with history of injection drug use at least once.
- Routine testing for asymptomatic patients for syphilis, Hepatitis B and C, human papilloma virus (HPV), herpes and trichomonas is not recommended. Pregnant adolescents may benefit from testing for some of these infections as part of their prenatal care.
- All teens should be screened and counseled on high-risk behavior that leads to the acquisition of any of these infections.
- Primary prevention of HPV, Hepatitis A and B through vaccination should be encouraged.

Adolescent testing for *N. gonorrheae*, *C. trachomatis*, and other vaginitis

Adolescents present a challenging population to screen utilizing traditional pelvic examination. While in the adult the practice of an internal vaginal examination is acceptable, for many teenagers this practice is unacceptable, threatening, and may prevent them from seeking medical care for fear of the examination. The available alternative methods of screening for certain STI using alternative body fluids and collection techniques has allowed for an increase in the utilization of screening services.

NAATs has increased the ability not only to detect, in a reliable manner, organisms that are present in low concentrations, but has also allowed the use of other body fluids instead of endocervical or urethral specimen collection. NAATs has been approved for the use in urine specimens in men and women, but proper specimen collection is critically important (Table 2.2).

As technology has improved, new specimen collection kits are available that allow patients to undergo self-testing by collecting their own vaginal specimen. The sensitivity of self-vaginal swab testing is comparable to urine or endocervical swabs and facilitates patient screening. Recent data suggests that adolescents prefer this method, which may potentially increase the effectiveness of the screening programs. As the technology improves, self-testing for other pathogens such as herpes, trichomonas, and bacterial vaginosis may become available.

The use of NAAT technology for nongenital sites has not undergone FDA validation, but the CDC recommends its use in those centers where a validation study has been done with their technique. Further information on laboratory requirements needed to fulfill validation can be found at www.cdc.gov/std.

In some cases, using point-of-care testing for certain infectious agents is feasible and cost effective. For example, traditional testing for *T. vaginalis* or bacterial vaginosis involves a pelvic examination, preparation of a wet mount, and direct observation under the microscope. This traditional point-of-care test has poor reliability and interobserver accuracy. Most studies would quote a sensitivity of 30–60% for either condition, making the diagnosis difficult. New rapid DNA-based technology (15 minutes) has increased the accuracy of the test without the need for visual direct interpretation with sensitivities of 95% and specificities close to 100%. Utilization of these techniques in the office may increase accuracy in the diagnosis of these conditions and improve treatment at the time of the visit.

Management of specific prevalent infections

The treatment of specific pathogens is described in other chapters, but special considerations in children and adolescents will be reviewed in this section to facilitate the practitioners' management of some of these conditions, as well as serving as a quick reference for agents and dosing.

Herpes simplex virus

Neonatal herpes: patients with potential exposure during birth to maternal herpes genital infection should be managed in conjunction with a pediatric infectious disease specialist. The use of intravenous acyclovir on suspected or diagnosed cases post-delivery is recommended at a dose of 20 mg/kg every 8 hours for 14–21 days, depending on the location of the infection.

Diseases characterized by urethritis and cervicitis

Chlamydia treatment in adolescents and children over the age of 8 follows the same guidelines as the adult. In children, once again, management in collaboration with child protective services is critically important to assure a thorough and

Table 2.2. Urine specimen collection requirements

- Allow one hour from the last void.
- Not a clean catch specimen.
- Collect the first 5–10 mL (max) of urine in a sterile container.
- May be left for 24 hours at room temperature.

proper sexual abuse evaluation. Regimens effective for treatment include:

- Recommended regimen for children who weigh less than 45 kg: Erythromycin base or ethylsuccinate 50 mg/kg/day orally divided into 4 doses daily for 14 days.
- Recommended regimen for children who weigh 45 kg or more than 45 kg but who are less than 8 years of age: Azithromycin 1 g orally in a single dose.

Gonorrhea treatment in adolescents and children who weigh more than 45 kg is the same as the adult. In 2010, the CDC increased the dose of ceftriaxone to 250 mg IM single dose to increase its efficacy. Because of an increase in resistant strains, the use of fluoroquinolones is no longer indicated.

- Recommended regimen for children who weigh less than 45 kg: ceftriaxone 125 mg IM single dose.

Pelvic inflammatory disease (PID) treatment guidelines in adolescents are the same as for adults. Although the incidence of PID in children is very low, it does occur and may have an origin predominantly in endogenous flora. Of importance in this age group is the need for early diagnosis and the aggressive treatment of suspected cases. The long-term effects related to infertility secondary to tubal occlusion, especially with chlamydia, make this intervention a very important healthcare issue. Patients suspected of having PID should be treated and followed carefully, and frequently, to document the effectiveness of treatment. The results of the testing collected at the time of diagnosis should be followed and patients counseled appropriately about the results. Adolescents are a group with a significant risk of noncompliance with medical treatment and sometimes qualify for intrahospital management of their disease rather than as an outpatient, although this "requirement" has been removed from the formal CDC recommendations for PID treatment.

Patients who have been treated for gonorrhea or chlamydia may not require a "test of cure" (repeat NAAT testing at 4 weeks post-treatment) unless they are pregnant, there is a suspicion of reinfection, noncompliance, or persistence of symptoms. Patient with high-risk behavior and frequent partner change may benefit from testing for these infections every 6 months, or with every new partner. If a "test of cure" is performed, sufficient time should be allowed for the infectious material to dissolve, and should not be performed sooner than 4 weeks after treatment to prevent false-positive testing from dead organisms being detected by the highly sensitive NAAT methodology.

Conclusion

Caring for young patients requires a different set of skills than those used for adults. Concentrating in minimizing trauma and maximizing education should be the main focus of all those involved in the care of children and adolescents. Patience, appropriate documentation, and confidentiality play mayor roles in the successful examination of this population. Using alternative fluid testing for screening, such as urine, may improve compliance with future reproductive healthcare. Utilizing these techniques and the resources listed in the bibliography section, may allow the providers to perform the screening and treatment of these patients.

Bibliography

ACOG. *Tool Kit for Teen Care* (2nd edn.). American College of Obstetricians and Gynecologists, Washington, D.C., 2010.

Changes in the 2010 STD Treatment Guidelines: *What Adolescent Health Care Providers Should Know from the American College of Obstetricians and Gynecologists.* Adolescent Healthcare Division. Accessed on 5/11/2011 at: http://www.acog.org/departments/dept_notice.cfm?recno=7&bulletin=5545

Finkel MA, Giardino AP. (eds.). *Medical Examination of Child Sexual Abuse: A Practical Guide* (2nd edn.). Sage Publications: Thousand Oaks, CA, 2002; pp. 46–64.

Lara-Torre E. The physical examination in pediatric and adolescent patients. *Clinic Obstet Gynecol* 2008; **51**: 205–213.

McCann JJ, Kerns DL. *The Anatomy of Child and Adolescent Sexual Abuse: A CD-ROM Atlas/Reference.* MO, Intercort, Inc.: St. Louis, 1999.

North American Society of Pediatric and Adolescent Gynecology at www.naspag.org.

Pokorny SF, Stormer J: A traumatic removal of secretions from the prepubertal vagina. *Am J Obstet Gynecol* 1987; **156**: 581–582.

Sanfilippo JS, Lara-Torre E, Edmonds K, Templemand C (eds.). *Clinical Pediatric and Adolescent Gynecology*. Informa Healthcare USA, Inc., New York, NY, 2009.

Sanfilippo JS, Lara-Torre E. Adolescent gynecology. *Clinical Expert Series: Obstet Gynecol* 2009; **113**: 935–947.

Sexually Transmitted Diseases Treatment Guidelines 2010. MMWR December 17, 2010. Accessed on 5/11/2011 from http://www.cdc.gov/std/treatment/2010/default.htm

Cervicitis and Pelvic Inflammatory Disease

Oluwatosin Jaiyeoba and David E. Soper

Department of Obstetrics and Gynecology, Medical University of South Carolina, Charleston, SC, USA

Introduction

Cervicitis is an inflammatory process primarily affecting the columnar epithelial cells of the endocervical glands, but may also cause visible changes of the ectocervix, whose squamous epithelium is contiguous with that of the vagina. Two major diagnostic characteristics associated with cervicitis are purulent or mucopurulent endocervical exudate and sustained endocervical bleeding on gentle introduction of a cotton swab into the cervical os (also referred to as cervical friability). Gonorrhea and chlamydia infections account for less than one-half of cervicitis cases and others are referred to as nongonococcal, nonchlamydial cervicitis. Other pathogens that have been implicated include *Mycoplasma genitalium*, bacterial vaginosis, herpes simplex virus (HSV) and *Trichomonas vaginalis*. Cervicitis can be considered as a continuum with upper genital infection or pelvic inflammatory disease (PID) which is an infection-induced inflammation of the upper genital tract that includes endometritis, salpingitis, pelvic peritonitis, and/or a tubo-ovarian abscess (TOA). Acute PID is associated with significant sequelae including tubal factor infertility, ectopic pregnancy and chronic pelvic pain. To ameliorate these adverse outcomes, an approach to its diagnosis must promote the ability to intervene with antimicrobial therapy early

on in the course of this ascending infection. It is less important to accurately determine where the patient may lie along the continuum of this ascending inflammatory process (cervicitis, endometritis, salpingitis, or peritonitis) and more important to empirically initiate an appropriate antibiotic regimen when the diagnosis is suspected.

Pathophysiology

The sexually transmitted microorganisms *Neisseria gonorrheae* and *Chlamydia trachomatis* have been isolated from the cervix, endometrium, and fallopian tube of women with mucopurulent cervicitis, histologically confirmed endometritis and visually confirmed salpingitis. They are universally accepted as etiologic agents of cervical and upper genital tract infections. Trichomonas, candida, and HSV can cause inflammation of the ectocervix. Conversely, *N. gonorrheae* and *C. trachomatis* infect only the glandular epithelium. Bacterial vaginosis is a complex alteration of the vaginal microflora in which the normal lactobacilli-dominant vaginal flora is replaced with an anaerobic-dominant microflora in association with increasing concentrations of *Gardnerella vaginalis* and genital mycoplasmas. The microbial milieu of bacterial vaginosis is associated with the

Sexually Transmitted Diseases, First Edition. Edited by Richard H. Beigi.
© 2012 John Wiley & Sons, Ltd. Published 2012 by John Wiley & Sons, Ltd.

elaboration of a variety of mucolytic proteinases that appear to degrade the mucous plug and the naturally occurring antimicrobials, e.g. secretory leukocyte protease inhibitor, that reside on the genital tract mucosa. This potentiates the development of cervical inflammation and may facilitate ascending infection by cervical and vaginal microorganisms, thus resulting in endometritis and salpingitis. "Bacterial vaginosis microorganisms," particularly anaerobic Gram-negative rods, are associated with upper genital tract inflammation. Bacterial vaginosis, therefore, not only facilitates ascending spread of vaginal microorganisms by interfering with the host's defenses but also provides an inoculum of potentially pathogenic microorganisms. Rarely, respiratory pathogens, e.g. *Hemophilus influenzae* and *Streptococcus pneumoniae*, can be isolated from the fallopian tubes of women with salpingitis.

Investigators have reported detection of *M. genitalium* from the endocervix or endometrium or both in 14% of women with nongonococcal, nonchlamydial PID, and the microorganism has been isolated from the fallopian tube of a patient with visually confirmed salpingitis. *M. genitalium*-associated PID appears to present with mild clinical symptoms similar to chlamydial PID. There is little to no long-term morbidity associated with cervicitis or endometritis without the concurrent association of salpingitis. Once infection-induced inflammation reaches the fallopian tube, epithelial degeneration and deciliation of ciliated cells occurs along the fallopian tube mucosa in association with a submucosal inflammatory cell infiltrate. There is an associated edema of the fallopian tube that augments the intraluminal agglutination that occurs with endosalpingitis and leads to clubbing of the involved fallopian tube(s). This leads to a dysfunctional, partially or totally obstructed fallopian tube causing infertility or ectopic pregnancy. Peritonitis is characterized by a fibrinoid exudate on the serosal surfaces of the uterus, tubes, and ovaries leading to an agglutination of the tubes, ovaries, bowel, and omentum to the pelvic structures and to each other. This agglutination matures into both filmy and thick pelvic adhesive disease, which is a well-known cause of pelvic pain.

★ TIPS & TRICKS

- Evaluation of both vaginal and endocervical secretions for inflammation is an important component of PID diagnosis.
- Placement of the mucopus on a slide that can be Gram stained will reveal the presence of an increased number of neutrophils (>30 per high-power field) in cervicitis.
- Cervicitis is commonly associated with bacterial vaginosis (BV), which, if not treated concurrently, leads to significant persistence of the symptoms and signs of cervicitis.
- Have a high index of suspicion for PID in women < 25 years old or with risk factors for STI who have pelvic pain
- Early initiation of oral antibiotics in mild-moderate PID improves compliance and ameliorates PID sequelae
- Patients with persistent pelvic pain and negative NAATS who are at "lower risk for PID" need to be ruled out for other causes of pelvic pain esp. endometriosis.
- Patients with clinically severe PID need imaging to consider the presence of a TOA.
- Most women with a TOA will respond to medical therapy alone but in some, surgery can be life saving.

Diagnosis

Cervicitis, although often asymptomatic, should be considered as part of the differential diagnosis of young women presenting with either an abnormal vaginal discharge or intermenstrual bleeding. Two major diagnostic signs characterize cervicitis: (1) a purulent or mucopurulent endocervical exudate visible in the endocervical canal or on an endocervical swab specimen (commonly referred to as mucopurulent cervicitis), and (2) sustained endocervical bleeding easily induced by gentle passage of a cotton swab through the cervical os. Either or both signs might be present.

The diagnosis of PID is usually clinical, as shown in Figure 3.1 and PID should be considered in sexually active women with or without lower abdominal pain and symptoms noted in

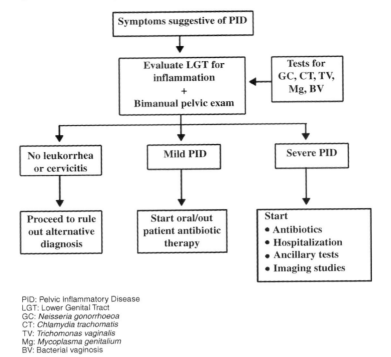

PID: Pelvic Inflammatory Disease
LGT: Lower Genital Tract
GC: *Neisseria gonorrhoeoa*
CT: *Chlamydia trachomatis*
TV: *Trichomonas vaginalis*
Mg: *Mycoplasma genitalium*
BV: Bacterial vaginosis

Figure 3.1. Flow chart showing clinical diagnosis of PID.

Table 3.1. An assessment of risk for a sexually transmitted infection (STI) enhances the specificity of the above presenting symptoms (Table 3.1); however, women without such risk factors should still have the diagnosis considered, given that many will not be accurate in believing that they reside in a mutually monogamous sexual relationship. Abdominal tenderness may

Table 3.1. Symptoms in women with clinically suspected pelvic inflammatory disease

---

Abdominal pain

Abnormal discharge

Intermenstrual bleeding

Postcoital bleeding

Fever

Urinary frequency

Low back pain

Nausea/vomiting

not be present in many women with PID, particularly if peritonitis is not present or the patient has endometritis without salpingitis. A bimanual pelvic examination may reveal pelvic organ tenderness, uterine tenderness in the case of endometritis, and adnexal tenderness in the case of salpingitis. Cervical motion tenderness is another common finding in women with PID. The Centers for Disease Control and Prevention (CDC) recommends empiric treatment for PID in sexually active young women (25 years old or younger) and other women at risk of STI (multiple sex partners or history of STI) if they are experiencing pelvic or lower abdominal pain, if no cause for the illness other than PID can be identified, and if one or more of the following is appreciated on bimanual pelvic examination: cervical motion tenderness, uterine tenderness, or adnexal tenderness. The limitation of this approach is that it fails to discriminate between the differential diagnoses of acute pelvic pain in reproductive-aged women. For this reason, the lower genital tract needs to be assessed for signs of inflammation.

The cervical canal should be examined for the presence of yellow or green mucopus and friability. Microscopy of the vaginal secretions should be performed looking for leukorrhea (more than 1 leukocyte per epithelial cell). Evaluation for bacterial vaginosis (vaginal pH, clue cells, and whiff test) and trichomonas vaginitis is in order. Finally, a nucleic acid amplification test (NAAT) for *N. gonorrheae* and *C. trachomatis* should be performed. If the cervix is normal and no white blood cells are noted during microscopy of the vaginal secretions, an alternative diagnosis should be investigated since this reliably excludes (negative predictive value 94.5%) upper genital tract infection. Because the sensitivity of microscopy to detect *T. vaginalis* is relatively low (approximately 50%), symptomatic women with cervicitis and negative microscopy for trichomonads require further testing (i.e. culture or polymerase chain reaction (PCR) method). Of note, NAAT for *C trachomatis* and *N. gonorrheae* can be performed on urine, vaginal, or cervical samples.

Other ancillary tests (Table 3.2) that can be useful in diagnosing PID include a complete blood count, erythrocyte sedimentation rate (ESR) or C-reactive protein (CRP). These tests are recommended for patients with clinically severe PID. Imaging studies are most helpful when ruling out competing differential diagnoses such as the use of pelvic ultrasonography to rule out symptomatic ovarian cysts and computed tomography (CT) to rule out appendicitis. Pelvic sonography has limited sensitivity for the diagnosis of PID, but the specific finding of thickened fluid-filled tubes by ultrasonography supports the diagnosis of upper genital tract inflammation. Pelvic sonography should be ordered in patients requiring hospitalization or those with a pelvic mass. If TOA is noted, a transvaginal ultrasound is the most cost-effective imaging to allow percutaneous drain placement. However, many interventional radiologists will prefer CT to guide drain placement.

It is less important to accurately determine where the patient may lie along the continuum of this ascending inflammatory process (cervicitis, endometritis, salpingitis, or peritonitis) and more important to empirically initiate an appropriate antibiotic regimen when the diagnosis is suspected.

Table 3.2. Signs and tests to Increase the specificity of a diagnosis of salpingitis

An additional sign and abnormal laboratory tests increase the specificity of the diagnosis of PID:

- Oral temperature 101 °F (>38.3 °C)
- Elevated C-reactive protein (CRP)
- Laboratory documentation of cervical *N. gonorrheae* or *C. trachomatis*.

The most specific criteria for the diagnosis of PID include:

- Endometrial biopsy with histologic evidence of endometritis
- Transvaginal sonography or MRI showing thickened, fluid filled tubes with or without free pelvic or tubo-ovarian complex or dopplers studies suggesting pelvic infection (tubal hyperemia)
- Laparoscopic abnormalities consistent with PID.

SCIENCE REVISITED

- Remember PID is an ascending infection and polymicrobial in nature.
- It is less important to accurately determine where the patient may lie along the continuum of the ascending inflammatory process (Cervicitis, endometritis, salpingitis, or peritonitis) than to empirically initiate an appropriate antibiotic regimen when the diagnosis is suspected.

Neisseria gonorrheae

Gonorrhea is the second most commonly reported bacterial STI in the United States. It accounts for approximately 300,000 new cases annually and probably an equal number of cases that are unreported. It is a major cause of urethritis in men and cervicitis in women; the latter can result in PID, infertility, ectopic pregnancy, and chronic pelvic pain if untreated.

The epidemiology of gonococcal infections in the United States has undergone changes in recent years. According to the CDC, there were 301,174 reported cases of gonorrhea in 2009, a 10% decline from the past year. Despite the decline, major racial disparities still remain; gonorrhea infection is 20 times higher in blacks compared to whites. Reasons for the racial disparity in gonorrhea rates are not well understood but probably include differences in health services access and utilization, geographic clustering of populations, socioeconomic factors, and sex partner choices. The highest reported rates of gonococcal infection are seen among adolescents and young adults, minorities, and persons living in the southeastern United States. Risk factors include new sex partner or multiple sex partners, being unmarried, young age, minority ethnicity, low educational and socioeconomic levels, substance abuse, and previous gonorrhea infection.

There is concern regarding the increase in antibiotic resistance in the treatment of gonococcal infections. Quinolones are no longer recommended in the United States for the treatment of gonorrhea and, more recently, resistance to cephalosporins is becoming an important problem in several parts of the country. The potential emergence and spread of both oral and parenteral cephalosporin-resistance in *N. gonorrheae* (Ceph-R NG) needs to be monitored and action needs to be taken to avoid a major public health problem. Although cephalosporins remain an effective treatment for gonococcal infections, patients with treatment failure should have *N. gonorrheae* culture and antimicrobial susceptibility testing performed to ascertain cephalosporin resistance.

Neisseria gonorrheae, a nonmotile, nonspore-forming Gram-negative dipolococcus, tends to cause an intense acute inflammatory reaction, often producing symptoms shortly after infection. On the other hand, approximately 50% of women with a gonococcal infection may remain asymptomatic, making screening at risk populations important for infection detection and upper genital tract disease prevention. Infection with *N. gonorrheae* encompasses four specific stages: attachment to the mucosal cell surface, local penetration or invasion, local proliferation, and local inflammatory response or dissemination. Most common site of mucosal infection with *N. gonorrheae* is the cervix. Symptomatic women may have vaginal pruritus and/or a mucopurulent discharge. Infection in women can present as cervicitis, urethritis, or anorectal infection. PID, an ascending infection, is a complication of untreated gonococcal infection, which can lead to infertility.

Diagnosis can be performed using culture, nucleic acid hybridization tests, and nucleic acid amplification tests. Culture and nucleic hybridization tests require an endocervical specimen, while NAAT can be performed on endocervical swab, vaginal swab, or urine. Culture is required in cases of treatment failure as stated above in order to perform antimicrobial susceptibility testing. In order to maximize compliance, it is recommended that antibiotics for gonococcal infections be administered on site and the CDC recommends a combination therapy of a single dose of ceftriaxone 250 mg plus azithromycin or doxycycline as first-line therapy. The ceftriaxone dose recommended by the CDC provides sustained and high bactericidal levels in the blood. The 2010 CDC guidelines for the treatment of uncomplicated gonococcal infection are listed in Table 3.3. Pregnant women should get the same dose of ceftriaxone as nonpregnant women.

Chlamydia trachomatis

Chlamydia genital infection is the most common bacterial STI in the Unites States with the highest prevalence seen in persons aged 25 years and younger. The majority of the women are

Table 3.3. The CDC 2010 recommended regimens for uncomplicated gonococcal infection

Ceftriaxone 250 mg IM in a single dose
or, if not an option
Cefixime 400 mg orally in a single dose
Or
Single-dose injectible cephalosporin regimens
Plus
Azithromycin 1 g orally in a single dose
Or
Doxycycline 100 mg a day for 7 days

asymptomatic, thereby providing an ongoing reservoir for infection. Approximately 4 million cases of chlamydial infection occur annually in the United States with an overall prevalence of 5%, making this the most common STI and one of the leading causes of infertility in women. *C. trachomatis* and *N. gonorrheae* cause similar clinical syndromes, but chlamydia infections tend to have fewer acute manifestations and more significant long-term complications.

The highest rates are in African-American women and the overall infection rate is higher in women than in men, with rates 4 times higher in females. Risk for infection include being young or adolescent, having new or multiple sex partners, inconsistent use of barrier contraception, cervical ectopy, unmarried status, history of prior STI, and lower socioeconomic class or education not beyond high school. Clinical manifestation includes cervicitis, dysuria-pyuria syndrome, perihepatitis, and PID.

C. trachomatis is a small obligate intracellular bacterial pathogen that has a unique biphasic life cycle. The infectious form (elementary body) is taken into the columnar cells where it converts into the metabolically active form (reticulate body). After this process, the host cell is sacrificed and an infectious elementary body is released to infect other host cells. Despite this process, previous infection with *C. trachomatis* does not provide protective immunity. *C. trachomatis* can be harbored, produce significant upper genital tract damage, and be transmitted despite being asymptomatic (nearly 70% of the time) in women. Mucosal infection induces a local inflammatory response which is characterized by lymphocytes and mononuclear cells.

Diagnosis can be performed using urine, self-collected vaginal swabs, or an endocervical swab. NAAT has good sensitivity (85%) and specificity (94–99.5%) for endocervical and urethral samples when compared with urethral culture. It is the preferred test and most commonly used method of diagnosis. It consists of amplifying *C. trachomatis* DNA or RNA sequences using PCR, transcription-mediated amplication (TMA), or strand displacement amplification (SDA).

The 2010 CDC guidelines for the treatment of chlamydia infection are listed in Table 3.4. Doxycycline, ofloxacin, and levofloxacin are contra-

Table 3.4. The CDC 2010 recommended regimens for chlamydial infection

Azithromycin 1 g orally in a single dose
Or
Amoxicillin 500 mg orally 3 times a day for 7 days
Alternative regimens
Erythromycin base 500 mg orally 4 times a day for 7 days
Or
Erythromycin base 250 mg orally 4 times a day for 14 days
Or
Erythromycin ethylsuccinate 800 mg orally 4 times a day for 7 days
Or
Erythromycin ethylsuccinate 400 mg orally 4 times a day for 14 days

indicated in pregnant women; however, azithromycin is safe and effective. CDC recommends repeat testing 3 weeks after completion of therapy for all pregnant women to document the eradication of chlamydia. Pregnant women diagnosed and treated for chlamydia in the first trimester should be retested 3 weeks later to document eradication and also retested 3 months after treatment. Pregnant women who are at increased risk of reinfection should be retested during the third trimester to prevent neonatal chlamydial infection.

Trichomonas vaginalis

T. vaginalis may be identified in vaginal secretions by using wet preparation, but this is only 35–80% sensitive compared to culture. The sensitivity of wet preparation is highly dependent on the microscopist and the prompt transport and laboratory processing of samples before organisms become lysed or lose motility. Diagnostic techniques include fluorescent antibody enzyme-linked immunosorbent assay and hybridization test, which have reported sensitivities between 70 and 90%. Culture in microaerophilic conditions is estimated to be 85 to 95% sensitive and has been considered the "gold standard" for diagnosis. PCR targeting the beta-tubulin genes of *T. vaginalis* has been developed for the detection of the organism in vaginal swab samples. PCR results are available in 2–3 days and provide the highest sensitivity of 97% with a specificity of 98%.

Mycoplasma genitalium

This is a fastidious microorganism with no cell wall. It is an established causative organism in nongonococcal urethritis (NGU) in men and has been implicated in mucopurulent cervicitis, endometritis, and salpingitis in women. Although commercial testing for this microorganism is not readily available, there is ongoing research to provide a PCR test for the detection of *M. genitalium* in a clinical setting.

Treatment

Treatment of cervicitis and PID should take into account the short-term goals of clinical and microbiological cure and the long-term goals of prevention of infertility, ectopic pregnancy, recurrent infection, and chronic pelvic pain. Optimal antimicrobial regimens should be well tolerated with little to no gastrointestinal side effects and tailored for compliance. Oral therapy is preferred over parenteral therapy in most clinical scenarios for reasons of convenience and cost, as well as to avoid the pain of needle injection.

⚠ CAUTION

- Diagnosis of PID can be difficult and often missed even by astute clinicians based on the wide variation in symptoms and signs.
- Early initiation of antibiotics in cervicitis or suspected PID is key.
- Tubo-ovarian abscess (TOA) warrants hospitalization and IV antibiotics.
- Ruptured TOA is a gynecologic surgical emergency!

Cervicitis

Presumptive treatment for *C. trachomatis* should be provided for women at increased risk of STIs, especially if follow-up cannot be ensured. Concurrent treatment for *N. gonorrheae* is indicated if the prevalence of this infection is greater than 5% in the population. It is also known that up to 27% of these women with cervicitis will have histologic evidence of endometritis; therefore, we must be confident that antibiotic therapy for cervicitis will not only treat the potential pathogens noted but also result in a resolution of endometritis if present. The CDC recommended presumptive therapy for cervicitis is single-dose azithromycin 1 g or doxycycline 100 mg orally twice daily for 7 days (Table 3.5), and the recommended gonococcal and chlamydial therapy are listed in Tables 3.3 and 3.4. Metronidazole may be withheld if no evidence of BV or *T. vaginalis* is present. The treatment of women diagnosed with gonorrhea and/or chlamydia should be based on CDC recommendations (Tables 3.3 and 3.4).

Follow-up

Women with persistent cervicitis should be re-evaluated for possible re-exposure to an STI. If symptoms persist, women should be instructed to return for re-evaluation as women with documented chlamydial or gonococcal infections have a high rate of reinfection within 6 months after treatment. Repeat testing is recommended 3–6 months after treatment for all women, regardless of whether their sex partners were treated.

Management of sex partners

Sex partners should be notified and examined if chlamydia, gonorrhea, or trichomoniasis was treated in the index patient and these partners should be treated for the STI for which the index patient received treatment. Patients and their partners should abstain from sexual intercourse

Table 3.5. The CDC 2010 recommended regimens for presumptive treatment of cervicitis[a]

Azithromycin 1 g orally in a single dose
Or
Doxycycline 100 mg orally twice a day for 7 days

[a] Consider concurrent treatment for gonococcal infection if prevalence of gonorrhea is high in the patient population under assessment.

until therapy is completed (7 days after a single-dose regimen or after completion of a 7-day regimen).

The process of treating sex partners without their mandatory prior examination is called Expedited Partner Therapy (EPT). EPT is the clinical practice of treating sex partners of persons with STIs by providing prescriptions or medications to the patient to take to her partner without the healthcare provider first examining the partner. In early studies, EPT appears to reduce the rates of persistent or recurrent gonorrhea or chlamydial infection and increases the proportion of partners treated per index patient report. Prior to the offer of EPT, providers should be aware of their state laws governing this practice.

Mild to moderate PID

These patients can safely be treated as outpatients. The CDC recommended regimens allows substitution of cefoxitin with other extended spectrum cephalosporins, such as ceftriaxone, ceftizoxime, cefotaxime. CDC also allows the clinician discretion to extend the anaerobic coverage by prescribing oral metronidazole in addition to the above mentioned doxycycline (Table 3.6).

Several quinolone antimicrobials (moxifloxacin, ciprofloxacin, and ofloxacin) alone or in combination with other agents have been studied and shown to be effective in the treatment of PID. However, ciprofloxacin appeared to be less effective in clearing bacterial vaginosis-associated microorganisms from the endometrium despite the patient's clinical cure. In addition, due to increasing *N. gonorrheae* resistance, *quinolone use is no longer recommended* for the treatment of *N. gonorrheae* in the United States and therefore cannot be considered a primary monotherapy option for the treatment of PID in areas with quinolone-resistant *N. gonorrheae* (QRNG). In areas where QRNG is uncommon, moxifloxacin is an antibiotic that can be considered for the treatment of acute PID. In three randomized-controlled trials, moxifloxacin has been found to be an effective and well-tolerated oral treatment in women with acute PID.

While doxycycline is the most commonly prescribed antibiotic in conjunction with cephalosporin therapy for PID, azithromycin provides

Table 3.6. The CDC 2010 recommended oral regimen (mild–moderate PID)

Ceftriaxone 250 mg IM in a single dose
Plus
Doxycycline 100 mg orally twice a day for 14 days
with or without
Metronidazole 500 mg orally twice a day for 14 days
Or
Cefoxitin 2 g IM in a single dose and probenecid 1 g orally administered concurrently in a single dose
Plus
Doxycycline 100 mg orally twice a day for 14 days
with or without
Metronidazole 500 mg orally twice a day for 14 days
Or
Other parenteral third-generation cephalosporin (e.g. ceftizoxime or cefotaxime)
Plus
Doxycycline 100 mg orally twice a day for 14 days
with or without
Metronidazole 500 mg orally twice a day for 14 days

excellent coverage of chlamydia and moderate-to-good coverage for a range of aerobic and anaerobic bacteria, including Gram-negative anaerobes. Azithromycin has been shown to be an effective alternative to doxycycline for the treatment of PID in prospective studies. In the macaque animal model, azithromycin was more effective in eradicating chlamydial organisms from the upper and lower reproductive tract tissues than doxycycline, and also exerted a significant anti-inflammatory effect. Azithromycin advantages over doxycycline include single-dose administration for chlamydial infection (azithromycin 1 g orally in a single dose versus doxycycline 100 mg orally twice a day for 7 days) and fewer side effects. In the treatment of mild to

Table 3.7. Criteria for hospitalization in women with pelvic inflammatory disease

- Surgical emergencies (e.g. appendicitis) cannot be excluded
- Patient is pregnant
- Patient does not respond clinically to oral antibiotic therapy
- Patient is unable to follow or tolerate an outpatient oral regimen
- Patient has severe illness, nausea and vomiting or high fever
- Patient has a tubo-ovarian abscess

moderate PID, azithromycin is administered as 500 mg orally (day 1) followed by 250 mg orally daily for a total of 7 days. *N. gonorrheae* resistance to azithromycin has been reported and the higher 2-g dose recommended to treat this pathogen is associated with significant gastrointestinal side effects, which complicates this approach. An alternative dosing schedule is single-dose azithromycin 1 g orally, repeated in 7 days. Both doxycycline and azithromycin should be used in conjunction with a cephalosporin.

Severe PID and tubo-ovarian abscess

Women with clinically severe PID, or meeting the criteria noted in Table 3.7, or both, should be considered for hospitalization and inpatient parenteral therapy. These patients most likely have nonchlamydial polymicrobial PID or, less commonly, acute gonococcal PID. Imaging should be considered in hospitalized patients to evaluate for other diseases and or abscess. Women hospitalized with severe PID may have TOA, and imaging with pelvic ultrasonography, magnetic resonance imaging (MRI), or CT is recommended. The most severe form of clinical PID-ruptured TOA should be considered in patients with PID presenting with an acute abdomen and signs of septic shock. Tubo-ovarian abscesses in patients undergoing medical management of PID may rupture and require emergent surgical therapy (Figures 3.2 and 3.3). Although 75% of women with TOAs will respond to antibiotic therapy alone, some will fail to respond and require surgical intervention.

The need for surgical intervention is related to the diameter of the TOA: 60% of those with abscesses 10 cm or greater; 30% of those with abscesses 7–9 cm; and only 15% of those with abscesses 4–6 cm. Patients, who fail to respond to antibiotic treatment within 48 to 72 hours, as characterized by persistent fever or increasing leukocytosis, should be considered for surgical drainage. Drainage of the TOA can be performed by laparotomy, laparoscopy, or image-guided percutaneous routes. Surgical exploration with extirpation of the involved adnexa and drainage of purulent loculations can

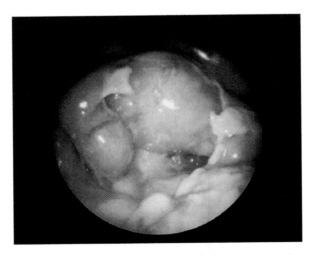

Figure 3.2. Laparoscopy visually confirms the presence of edematous, erythematous fallopian tubes and thick, sticky purulent exudates covering the uterus, tubes, and ovaries.

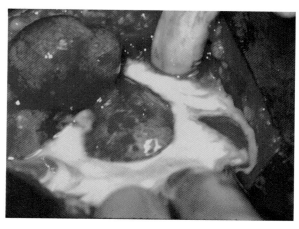

Figure 3.3. Exploratory laparotomy confirms the presence of copious purulent exudates covering the pelvic organs. There is associated hyperemia and edema of the pelvic organs documenting upper genital inflammation.

be lifesaving in women with a ruptured TOA, and a hysterectomy is not usually necessary.

Proper antimicrobial therapy of pelvic abscesses includes an antibiotic regimen with activity against anaerobic bacteria such as *Bacteroides fragilis* and *Prevatella bivius,* which produce beta-lactamase. In addition, an antimicrobial regimen should have good coverage for *Escherichia coli,* which is a common and predominant isolate from patients with a ruptured TOA and a well-recognized cause of Gram-negative sepsis. Regimens recommended for this clinical scenario include the combination regimens of clindamycin with gentamicin, cefotetan or cefoxitin with doxycycline, and ampicillin/sulbactam with doxycycline (see Table 3.8). If a TOA is present, regimens should have the ability to penetrate abscess cavities while remaining stable in an acidic, hypoxic abscess environment. Although regimens containing an aminoglycoside have been used effectively in women with pelvic abscesses, this class of antibiotic has its activity significantly reduced at low pH, low oxygen tension, and in the presence of drug-binding purulent debris. An extended spectrum cephalosporin, e.g. ceftriaxone, may be a better choice to combine with either clindamycin or metronidazole in treating women with severe PID with or without a TOA. Not only do extended spectrum cephalosporins maintain their activity in an abscess environment, but they have a much high-

er serum level to minimum inhibitory concentration ratio than the aminoglycosides.

Clindamycin is actively transported into polymorphonuclear leukocytes and macrophages and is present in relatively high concentrations in experimental abscesses. Clindamycin is used in combination therapy for PID because of its activity against anaerobes, and it continues to be recommended in the treatment of PID on the basis of earlier studies and previously successful experiences, but resistance to clindamycin has been observed among isolates recovered from the lower genital tract. For the reasons noted above, we recommend metronidazole or clindamycin in combination with ceftriaxone as a regimen of choice. Other antimicrobials with similar broad spectrum coverage and activity within the hostile environment of the abscess include beta-lactam agents with beta-lactamase inhibitors (e.g. ampicillin/sulbactam, ticarcillin/clavulanate, and piperacillin/tazobactam) and the carbapenems (e.g. ertapenem, merepenem, and imipenem/cilistatin). Finally, for those women with an immediate hypersensitivity to penicillin, we would recommend the combination of a quinolone (e.g. ciprofloxacin or levofloxacin) plus metronidazole. It would be important to test for *N. gonorrheae* by culture in these patients as susceptibility to quinolones would need to be ascertained. Patients admitted with severe PID and/or a TOA should be discharged on a

Table 3.8. The CDC 2010 recommended parenteral regimen A

Cefotetan 2 g IV every 12 hours
Or
Cefoxitin 2 g IV every 6 hours
Plus
Doxycycline 100 mg orally or IV every 12 hours
Recommended parenteral regimen B
Clindamycin 900 mg IV every 8 hours
Plus
Gentamicin loading dose IV or IM (2 mg/kg of body weight), followed by a maintenance dose (1.5 mg/kg) every 8 hours. Single daily dosing (3–5 mg/kg) can be substituted.
Alternative parenteral regimens
Ampicillin/sulbactam 3 g IV every 6 hours
Plus
Doxycycline 100 mg orally or IV every 12 hours

broad-spectrum oral antimicrobial regimen to complete a 14-day course. Recommended oral regimens for discharge include amoxicillin/clavulanate (875 mg twice daily) or the combination of trimethoprim/sulfamethoxazole (160/800 mg twice daily) and metronidazole (500 mg twice daily) due to the excellent polymicrobial coverage.

Sequelae

The sequelae associated with acute salpingitis are tubal factor infertility, ectopic pregnancy, chronic pelvic pain, and an increased risk of recurrent infection. When compared with healthy women in a control group or with women with a clinical diagnosis of PID but negative laparoscopic findings, women with laparoscopically confirmed acute salpingitis were more likely to be infertile, to develop an ectopic pregnancy, and to report chronic abdominal pain. Infertility was 2.6 times more common in those women who delayed seeking healthcare 3 or more days after the onset of abdominal pain. Infertility was also more common in women with increasing severity of acute salpingitis when laparoscopically graded. Finally, infertility increased with additional episodes of PID. Women with either laparoscopically or clinically diagnosed PID are at higher risk of chronic pelvic pain, defined as menstrual or nonmenstrual pain of at least 6-month duration. Furthermore, chronic pelvic pain is found in 18–75% of women with PID compared with only 5–25% of unaffected women.

Prevention

Methods for preventing the transmission of STI are well known. They include abstinence, reduction in the number of sex partners, and the consistent and correct use of contraceptives. Efforts to prevent PID must also address the earliest parts of this causal chain – that is, they must emphasize the primary prevention or early detection of infections of the lower genital tract. One study showed that a strategy of identifying, testing, and treating women at increased risk of cervical chlamydial infection can reduce the incidence of PID. The US Preventive Services Task Force (USPSTF) and the CDC recommend screening for chlamydia in sexually active women 25 years of age and younger as well as high-risk (multiple sex partners or a history of prior sexually transmitted disease or both) women over 25. The USPSTF also recommends that clinicians screen all sexually active women (including those who are pregnant) for gonorrhea infection if they are at increased risk for infection. Women under the age of 25 years are considered to be at highest risk for infection, and clinicians should also consider population-based risk factors and the local epidemiology of the disease. Finally, the sex partners of women with PID should be examined and treated for gonococcal and chlamydial infection regardless of the pathogens detected in the patient with PID. These male sex partners are commonly asymptomatic, but still have a strong likelihood of being infected.

Bibliography

Brunham RC, Paavonen J, Stevens CE, et al. Mucopurulent cervicitis – the ignored counterpart in women of urethritis in men. *New Engl J Med* 1984; **311**: 1–6.

Centers for Disease Control and Prevention 2009. Sexually transmitted diseases surveillance: gonorrhea. Available at: http://www.cdc.gov/STD/stats09/gonorrhea.htm.

Centers for Disease Control and Prevention. Cephalosporin susceptibility among *Neisseria gonorrheae* isolates – United States, 2000–2010. *MMWR* 2011; **60** (26): 873–877.

Centers for Disease Control and Prevention. Sexually transmitted diseases treatment guidelines, *MMWR* 2010; **59** (No. RR-12): 2010.

Eckert LO, Thwin SS, Hillier SL, et al. The antimicrobial treatment of subacute endometritis: a proof of concept study. *Am J Obstet Gynecol* 2004; **190**: 305–313.

Eschenbach DA, Hillier S, Critchlow C, et al. Diagnosis and clinical manifestations of bacterial vaginosis. *Am J Obstet Gynecol* 1988; **158**: 819–828.

Eschenbach DA, Wolner-Hanssen P, Hawes SE, et al. Acute pelvic inflammatory disease: associations of clinical and laboratory findings with laparoscopic findings. *Obstet Gynecol* 1997; **89** (2): 184–192.

Haggerty CL, Totten PA, Astete SG, et al. Failure of cefoxitin and doxycycline to eradicate endometrial *Mycoplasma genitalium* and the consequence for clinical cure of pelvic inflammatory disease. *Sex Transm Infect* 2008; **84**: 338–342.

Jacobson L and Westrom L. Objectivized diagnosis of acute pelvic inflammatory disease. *Am J Obstet Gynecol* 1969; **105**: 1088–1098.

Judlin P, Liao Q, Liu Z, et al. Efficacy and safety of moxifloxacin in uncomplicated pelvic inflammatory disease: the MONALISA study. *Br J Gynecol* 2010; 1111/j.1471-0528.2010.02687

Kiviat NB, Wolner-Hanssen P, Eschenbach DA, et al. Endometrial histopathology in patients with culture-proved upper genital tract infection and laparoscopically diagnosed acute salpingitis. *Am J Surg Pathol* 1990; **14** (2): 167–175.

Landers DV, Sweet RL. Current trends in the diagnosis and treatment of tuboovarian abscess. *Am J Obstet Gynecol* 1085; **151**: 1098–1110.

Ness RB, Soper DE, Holley RL, et al. Effectiveness of inpatient and outpatient treatment strategies for women with pelvic inflammatory disease: Results from the Pelvic Inflammatory Disease Evaluation and Clinical Health (PEACH) Randomized Trial. *Am J Obstet Gynecol* 2002; **186**: 929–937.

Schwebke JR, Schulien MB, Zajackowski M. Pilot study to evaluate the appropriate management of patients with coexisting bacterial vaginosis and Cervicitis. *Infect Dis Obstet Gynecol* 1995; **3**: 119–122.

Soper DE, Brockwell NJ, Dalton HP, Johnson D. Microbial etiology of urban emergency department acute salpingitis: treatment with ofloxacin. *Am J Obstet Gynecol* 1992; **167**: 653–660.

Soper DE, Brockwell NJ, Dalton HP, Johnson D. Observations concerning the microbial etiology of acute salpingitis. *Am J Obstet Gynecol* 1994; **170**: 1008–1014.

Thurman AR, Soper DE. Sequelae. In: *Pelvic Inflammatory Disease* (Sweet RL, Wiesenfeld HC, eds.). Boca Rotan, FL: Taylor & Francis, 2006; pp. 69–83.

Wiesenfeld HC, Hillier SL, Krohn MA, et al. Lower genital tract infection and endometritis: insight into subclinical pelvic inflammatory disease. *Obstet Gynecol* 2002; **100**: 456–463.

Workowski KA, Berman SM, Douglas JM. Emerging antimicrobial resistance in *Neisseria gonorrheae*: Urgent need to strengthen prevention strategies. *Ann Intern Med* 2008; **148**: 606–613.

Yudin MH, Hillier SL, Wiesenfeld HC, et al. Vaginal polymorphonuclear leukocytes and bacterial vaginosis as markers for histologic endometritis among women without symptoms of pelvic inflammatory disease. *Am J Obstet Gynecol* 2003; **188**: 318–233.

4

Genital Herpes Simplex Infections in Women

Carolyn Gardella

Department of Obstetrics and Gynecology, Division of Women's Health, University of Washington, Seattle and Department of Surgery, Division of Gynecology, Department of Veterans Affairs, Puget Sound Health Care System, Seattle, WA, USA

Epidemiology

Genital herpes simplex virus (HSV) infection is one of the most common sexually transmitted infections. Current estimates suggest that at least 45 million people older than age 12 are infected with genital herpes. This correlates to 1 out of 5 adolescents and adults, with the prevalence higher in women than in men. Although 1 in 5 persons has genital herpes, most people with genital herpes do not know that they carry the virus. A key contributor to transmission is lack of diagnosis of the infection. Seventy percent of genital herpes infections are transmitted by people who are asymptomatic or are unaware of their infections.

Although HSV-2 typically causes genital herpes, and HSV-1 orolabial herpes, an increasing proportion of genital herpes is caused by HSV-1. Among college students with newly diagnosed genital herpes, 80% were from HSV-1. The increase in genital HSV-1 is likely due to the increased practice of orogenital sex which is perceived by this age group as being a "safe" alternative to genital–genital sex.

Determining the HSV type that is causing genital herpes is useful for patient counseling. The frequency of genital reactivation is much less with HSV-1, which rarely recurs symptomatically or asymptomatically after the first year of infection. In contrast, genital HSV-2 continues to recur, often frequently, for many years.

Pathophysiology

HSV is a double-stranded DNA virus that can be identified as HSV-1 or HSV-2 by the glycoproteins in the lipid envelope. Transmission of HSV infections occurs through close contact with a person who is shedding virus at a peripheral site, mucosal surface, or in genital or oral secretions. Infection occurs by inoculation of HSV onto

---

Sexually Transmitted Diseases, First Edition. Edited by Richard H. Beigi.
© 2012 John Wiley & Sons, Ltd. Published 2012 by John Wiley & Sons, Ltd.

mucosal surfaces or cracks in the skin. The incubation period after exposure to HSV-1 or HSV-2 is 2 to 12 days. Once inoculated, HSV ascends peripheral sensory nerves and enters sensory or autonomic nerve root ganglia where latency is established. HSV reactivates and ascends the sensory nerve to mucosal surfaces, causing "viral shedding" that may be associated with herpetic lesions or may be asymptomatic. Infection is lifelong.

Type-specific antibodies to HSV develop within the first few weeks of infection and persist. Antibodies to HSV can be detected by most assays within 2–3 weeks after infection.

Clinical presentation

The classically described skin manifestations of genital herpes include grouped pustular or ulcerative lesions on the external genitalia. Typically the lesions start as papules or vesicles that rapidly spread, and coalesce into an ulcerative lesion. Lesions may last from days to weeks. Primary infection classically is associated with fever, headache, malaise and myalgias. This "classic" presentation occurs in the minority of cases.

Approximately 70% of newly acquired HSV infections among women are asymptomatic or unrecognized. The remaining 30% of women with new infections have clinical presentations that range from minimal lesions and mild discomfort to widespread genital lesions associated with severe local pain, dysuria, sacral parasthesia, tender regional lymph node enlargement, fever, malaise, and headache (see Figures 4.1–4.3).

Aseptic meningitis occurs less frequently, and disseminated disease is rare.

Similarly, reactivations of genital herpes are most commonly unrecognized. The spectrum of clinically evident episodes varies from very mild episodes to severe symptoms that can be clinically indistinguishable from a severe new infection (Figures 4.4 and 4.5). The clinical manifestations of genital herpes cannot be relied upon to diagnose infection or to differentiate a newly acquired infection from a reactivated infection. Approximately 90% of women with HSV-2 will have recurrences within the first 12 months after infection. The frequency of symptomatic recurrences gradually decreases over time. An average of four recurrences per year is common the first year after symptomatic genital HSV-2 infection. Approximately 60% of women with symptomatic HSV-1 infection will have a recurrence in the first year and most women have fewer than four symptomatic recurrences thereafter.

Providers should consider HSV when caring for women with subtle genital symptoms or with clinically unusual severe illness, especially in pregnancy. In all cases, the diagnosis of genital HSV infection requires laboratory confirmation, although antiviral therapy can be initiated, based on clinical presentation. The Centers for Disease Control and Prevention (CDC) recommend that both virologic tests and type-specific serologic tests for HSV be available in clinical settings that provide care for patients at risk for sexually transmitted infections.

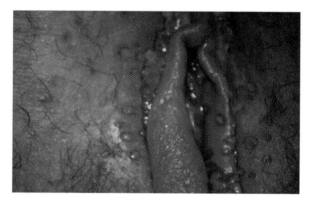

Figure 4.1. Typical severe manifestations of primary herpes simplex 2 viral infection with numerous simultaneous ulcers, vesicles, and confluent areas of ulceration.

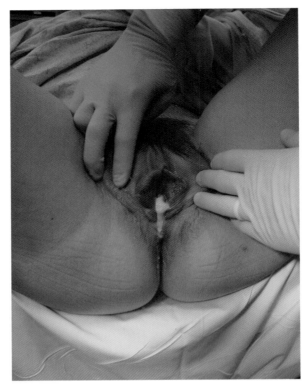

Figure 4.2. Ulcerations of primary herpes infection, with noted edema, confluent area of ulceration, and copious inflammatory discharge from primary herpes cervicitis.

Viral shedding

Asymptomatic viral shedding is an important cause of HSV transmission. Most episodes of sexual transmission occur during asymptomatic shedding. Genital HSV-2 is more likely to shed, and is more likely to shed without symptoms than genital HSV-1. The highest shedding rates occur in the first year of infection, and are widely variable among persons. Fifty percent of shedding episodes occur around symptomatic recurrences. Asymptomatic shedding can occur from any genital site including the cervix, vulva, perianal region in women and normal appearing penile skin or perianal region in men.

Diagnosis in women with genital lesions

The CDC recommends laboratory confirmation of a genital herpes diagnosis because clinical diagnosis is neither sensitive nor specific. Up to 20% of patients with an unconfirmed clinical

diagnosis of genital herpes are incorrectly diagnosed.

For women who present with a genital lesion, a specimen for viral culture can be collected and viral typing performed. The main disadvantages of viral culture are the difficulty in handling and the high false negative rate. Up to 75% of viral cultures from recurrent lesions are negative. Alternatively, polymerase chain reaction detects HSV DNA in lesions. It is 3–4 times more sensitive than viral culture and the specimen requires significantly less fastidious handling than a viral culture. PCR is becoming more readily available for routine clinical use, and is expected to replace viral culture in the near future. In all cases when virus is identified, either by culture or PCR, the specimen should be typed to determine if it is HSV-1 or HSV-2. This will facilitate safer-sex counseling and provide a prognosis for the clinical course. A negative HSV

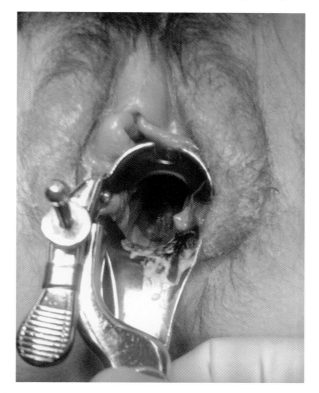

Figure 4.3. Primary herpes cervicitis (ectocervicitis). Note the erythematous and inflamed appearing cervix with purulent drainage.

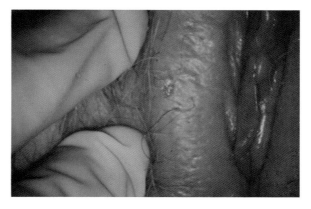

Figure 4.4. Solitary painful shallow ulceration typical of recurrent genital herpes.

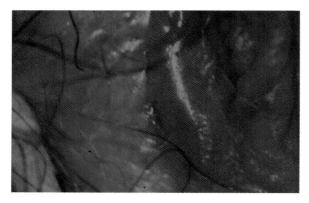

Figure 4.5. Subtle lateral recurrent genital herpes ulceration. Note that this lesion may not be appreciated on examination without careful observation.

culture or PCR result does not exclude a diagnosis of genital herpes.

When collecting a sample for viral culture or PCR, you are more likely to detect virus from a vesicle that you unroof than from an ulcer.

Diagnosis in women without lesions

In women who present with a history of lesions but none at the time of the clinical examination, serologic evaluation is the preferred diagnostic method. Only glycoprotein G-based type-specific antibody tests should be used so that HSV-1 and HSV-2 antibodies can be distinguished (Table 4.1). There are many HSV serologic tests commercially available that are not IgG based and are therefore not type specific. Therefore, it is important to order the test by name, or confirm that your lab is using an IgG-based test.

Table 4.1. Type-specific gG-based serology FDA approved commercial kits

Lab-based:
HerpeSelect 1 ELISA IgG
HerpeSelect 2 ELISA IgG
HerpeSelect 1 and 2 Immunoblot IgG
Point-of-care:
Biokit HSV-2 rapid test
Captia IgG enzyme immunoassay

SCIENCE REVISITED

Glycoprotein G is an epitope on HSV envelope that differs in HSV-1 and HSV-2.

☆ TIPS & TRICKS

All FDA approved tests have high sensitivity and acceptable specificity. However, the Focus ELISA tests require particular attention. In cases in which results of the Focus ELISA appear low positive, a confirmatory test such as the Biokit can be used. The manufacturer recommended interpretation of Focus HSV-2 EIA is: <0.9 is negative, 0.9–1.1 is indeterminate, >1.1 is positive. However, experts recommend confirmatory testing with Biokit for all sera with Focus ELISA values between 1.1 and 3.5.

The time necessary for serologic detection depends on the specific test being used. For Focus, it is a median of 20 days, and <20 days for the Biokit HSV-2 test. It generally requires 6 to 8 weeks for HSV IgG seroconversion to occur but can take up to 12 weeks or longer. If infection occurred during this time frame, retesting after 12 weeks is recommended if the initial serologic test is negative.

HSV-2 serology is also useful in patients with recurrent, undiagnosed or complicated genito-urinary symptoms as well as for patient with culture negative lesions or who have a clinical diagnosis of genital herpes without laboratory confirmation. All women requesting sexually transmitted infection screening, or requesting herpes testing, should have HSV serologic testing, as should any woman with a current or past sex partner with genital herpes. Those with positive HSV-2 serology should be counseled that they have genital herpes.

Interpretation of serologic test results

Using viral typing and type-specific serology, symptomatic genital herpes can be classified as new or recurrent. New infection is defined as isolation of HSV-1 or HSV-2 from genital secretions in the absence of concordant HSV antibodies in serum. Reactivation disease is characterized by isolation of HSV-1 or HSV-2 from the genital tract in the presence of HSV antibodies of the same serotype as the isolate.

Among asymptomatic persons, a woman with a positive HSV-2 serology should be counseled that she has genital herpes. Virtually all HSV-2 seropositive women will shed HSV-2 from the genital tract at some point. A woman whose HSV-1 serology is positive but asymptomatic at both sites is considered to have an HSV-1 infection of unknown site. If a new exposure occurred recently or she has been, or is symptomatic, an HSV-2 serology should be repeated in 8–12 weeks to allow time for seroconversion. If a patient is HSV seronegative, but recently exposed, consider repeating type-specific IgG serology in 8–12 weeks or reswab the genital lesions to establish definitive diagnosis (Table 4.2).

Management of genital herpes

Antiviral medications control the signs and symptoms of herpes when used to treat first clinical and recurrent episodes, or when used as daily suppressive therapy. The drugs do not eradicate latent virus; nor do they affect the risk, frequency, or severity of recurrence after the drug is discontinued.

First clinical episode of genital herpes

Newly acquired genital herpes can cause prolonged clinical illness with severe genital ulcerations and neurologic involvement. Even women with mild clinical manifestations initially can develop severe or prolonged symptoms. Therefore, CDC recommends that all patients with first episodes of genital herpes should receive antiviral therapy.

Centers for disease control treatment recommendations[1]

Acyclovir 400 mg orally 3 times a day for 7–10 days

or

Acyclovir 200 mg orally 5 times a day for 7–10 days

or

Famciclovir 250 mg orally 3 times a day for 7–10 days

[1]Treatment can be extended if healing is incomplete after 10 days of therapy.

or

Valacyclovir 1 g orally twice a day for 7–10 days

Severe disease

Some patient will have severe disease or complications such as disseminated infection, pneumonitis, hepatitis, or meningitis requiring hospitalization. For these patients, the CDC recommends intravenous acyclovir therapy. The recommended regimen is acyclovir 5–10 mg/kg IV every 8 hours for 2–7 days or until clinical improvement is observed, followed by oral antiviral therapy to complete at least 10 days of total therapy. An acyclovir dose adjustment is recommended for impaired renal function. For severe genital symptoms causing urinary retention, a foley catheter should be placed.

Analgesics, such as acetaminophen and ibuprofen, and warm water baths are recommended. Topical lidocaine can be beneficial in some cases but may cause local allergic reactions. Topical antiviral therapy is not effective and, therefore, not recommended.

Recurrent genital herpes

Antiviral therapy for recurrent genital herpes can be administered either as suppressive therapy to reduce the frequency of recurrences or episodically to shorten the duration of lesions. Taken daily, antiviral medication prevents approximately 80% of symptomatic genital recurrences. Suppressive therapy has the added benefit of reducing the risk of transmission to sex partners by reducing the risk of viral shedding, and decreasing the amount of virus shed if breakthrough shedding occurs. Suppressive therapy decreases transmission to uninfected sex partners by approximately 50%.

Effective episodic treatment of recurrent herpes requires the initiation of therapy within 1 day of lesion onset or during the prodrome that precedes some outbreaks. The patient should be provided with a supply of drug or a prescription for the medication with instructions to initiate treatment immediately when symptoms begin.

Viral resistance to acyclovir is very rare in immunocompetent persons, occurring in less than 1.0% of isolates. Among immunocompromised persons, however, the prevalence is approximately 7%.

Centers for disease control treatment recommendations[2]

Suppressive therapy

Acyclovir 400 mg orally twice a day
or
Famiciclovir 250 mg orally twice a day
or
Valacyclovir 500 mg orally once a day
or
Valacyclovir 1 g orally once a day

Episodic therapy

Acyclovir 400 mg orally 3 times a day for 5 days
or
Acyclovir 800 mg orally twice a day for 5 days
or
Acyclovir 800 mg orally 3 times a day for 2 days
or
Famciclovir 125 mg orally twice daily for 5 days
or
Famciclovir 1000 mg orally twice daily for 1 day
or
Famciclovir 500 mg once, followed by 250 mg twice daily for 2 days
or
Valacyclovir 500 mg orally twice a day for 3 days
or
Valacyclovir 1 g orally once a day for 5 days.

Counseling

Counseling regarding the diagnosis of genital herpes requires sensitivity to the fact that HSV is a life-long infection that may be perceived as stigmatizing to the patient. Psychological distress at the time of initial diagnosis is common, but usually self limited. A separate visit for counseling after the initial diagnosis is made often is helpful.

Common concerns include frequency of recurrences, sexual transmission, and impact on future pregnancy.

[2]Valacyclovir 500 mg once a day might be less effective than other valacyclovir or acyclovir dosing regimens in patients who have very frequent recurrences (i.e. >10 episodes per year).

Often women want to know when they acquired the virus, and have concerns about infidelity in current partnerships. Reassurance that most initial infections are asymptomatic and that she may have been infected remote from her first clinical episode, or that her current partner may have undiagnosed genital herpes, is helpful. She should be educated about the natural history of the disease, with emphasis on potential for recurrent episodes, asymptomatic viral shedding, and the risks of sexual transmission. She should be encouraged to inform her current sex partner and future partners prior to initiating a sexual relationship. To minimize, but not eliminate, the risk of transmission, they should not have sex when she has symptoms or prodromal symptoms, she can consider using daily antiviral suppressive therapy, and use male latex condoms consistently, both of which decrease transmission risk by about 50%.

Patients should receive information about suppressive and episodic therapy and the choice should take the frequency of recurrences, psychosocial distress, and partner susceptibility into consideration. If episodic therapy is preferred, women should have the medication on hand to initiate during prodrome or at the first appearance of lesions.

Sex partners of infected persons should be advised that they may be infected even if they do not have symptoms. Type-specific serologic testing of asymptomatic partners is recommended to determine if they already are HSV seropositive or if they are at risk of acquiring HSV.

The CDC recommends that the risk of neonatal herpes should be explained to all persons, including men. Pregnant women and women of childbearing age who have genital herpes should inform their providers who care for them during pregnancy, and those who will care for their newborn infant, about their infection. Pregnant women who are not known to be infected with HSV-2 should be advised to abstain from intercourse with men who have genital herpes during the third trimester of pregnancy. Pregnant women who are not known to be infected with HSV-1 should be counseled to avoid genital exposure to HSV-1 during the third trimester.

Written or web-based educational material should be provided to the patient. The American Social Health Association is one such excellent resource (ashastd.org).

HSV in pregnancy

Women who are shedding HSV from the genital tract at the time of labor are at risk of transmitting HSV to their neonates. Neonatal herpes is a rare but potentially devastating complication of genital herpes that presents within the first 28 days of life. Women with a newly acquired infection are at greatest risk (30–50%) of transmitting to the neonate, whereas women with a recurrent infection are at low, *but not nil*, risk of transmitting (1–3%). Women with recurrent infections have HSV antibodies that cross the placenta and decrease the risk of neonatal infection if exposed to HSV.

Table 4.2. Interpretation of type-specific serologic tests for herpes

HSV-1 Serology	HSV-2 Serology	Interpretation
−	+	Genital HSV-2 infection
+	−	HSV-1 infection; site unknown, unless a clear history of oral or genital herpes. Repeat HSV-2 serology in ≥8 weeks, if indicated, and reswab subsequent genital lesions.
+	+	Genital HSV-2 infection; probable orolabial HSV-1 infection
−	−	Repeat HSV-1 and HSV-2 serology in ≥8 weeks. Reswab subsequent genital lesions.

Table 4.3. Recommended doses of antiviral medications for herpes in pregnancy

Indication	Acyclovir	Valacyclovir
Primary or first-episode	400 mg orally, 3 times daily for 7–10 days	1 g orally, twice daily, for 7–10 days
Symptomatic recurrence	400 mg orally, 3 times daily for 5 days or 800 mg orally twice daily, for 5 days	500 mg orally, twice daily, for 3 days or 1 g orally, daily, for 5 days
Daily suppression	400 mg orally, 3 times daily, from 36 weeks until delivery	500 mg orally, twice daily, from 36 weeks until delivery
Severe or disseminated	5–10 mg/kg, intravenously, every 8 hours for 2–7 days, then oral therapy for primary infection to complete 10 days	

Adapted from: ACOG. Management of herpes in pregnancy. *ACOG Practice Bulletin* No. 82. American College of Obstetricians and Gynecologists. *Obstet Gynecol* 2007; **109**: 1233–1248.

For women with known genital herpes in pregnancy, the American College of Obstetricians and Gynecologists (ACOG) recommends antiviral therapy at the first clinical episode to reduce symptom duration. Additionally, ACOG recommends consideration of antiviral suppressive therapy for any woman with symptomatic genital herpes, to prevent genital lesions at the time of labor that would then require cesarean delivery (Table 4.3).

At the time of labor, all women should be questioned regarding symptoms of genital herpes, and the vulva, vagina, and cervix should be examined carefully for herpes lesions. If she does not have prodromal symptoms, or active lesions, vaginal birth is indicated. However, if she has symptoms or lesions, ACOG recommends a cesarean delivery to reduce neonatal exposure to genital herpes. Cesarean delivery significantly reduces, but does not completely eliminate, the risk of neonatal herpes. After delivery, the pediatrician should be informed of the maternal history to observe for early signs of neonatal infection.

EVIDENCE AT A GLANCE

Cochrane review of third trimester antiviral prophylaxis for preventing maternal genital herpes simplex virus recurrences and neonatal infection found that women who received antiviral prophylaxis were significantly less likely to have a recurrence of genital herpes at delivery (RR 0.28, 95% CI: 0.18–0.43), less likely to have a cesarean delivery for genital herpes (RR 0.30, 95% CI: 0.20–0.45), and less likely to have HSV detected at delivery (RR 0.14, 95% CI: 0.05–0.39). There was insufficient evidence to determine if antiviral prophylaxis reduced the risk of neonatal herpes.

Bibliography

ACOG. Gynecologic herpes simplex virus infections. *ACOG Practice Bulletin* No. 57. American College of Obstetricians and Gynecologists. *Obstet Gynecol* 2004; **104**: 1111–1118.

ACOG. Management of herpes in pregnancy. *ACOG Practice Bulletin* No. 82. American College of Obstetricians and Gynecologists. *Obstet Gynecol* 2007; **109**: 1489–1498.

Brown ZA, Gardella C, Wald A, Morrow RA, Corey L. Genital herpes complicating pregnancy [published erratum appears in *Obstet Gynecol* 2006; **107**: 428]. *Obstet Gynecol* 2005; **106**: 845–856.

Corey L, Wald A. Genital herpes. In: *Sexually Transmitted Diseases*, 4th edn. (Holmes KK, Sparling PF, Stamm WE, et al., eds.). New York: McGraw-Hill Medical, 2008; pp. 399–437.

Corey L, Wald A. Maternal and neonatal herpes simplex virus infections. *New Engl J Med* 2009; **361**: 1376–1385.

Corey L, Wald A, Patel R, Sacks SL, Tring SK, Warren T, et al. Once-daily valacyclovir to reduce the risk of transmission of genital herpes. Valacyclovir HSV Transmission Study Group. *New Engl J Med* 2004; **350**: 11–20.

Hollier LM, Wendel GD. Third trimester antiviral prophylaxis for preventing maternal genital herpes simplex virus (HSV) recurrences and neonatal infection. *Cochran Database Syst Rev* 2008 Jan; **(1)**: CD004946.

Wald A, Langenberg AG, Link K, et al. Effect of condoms on reducing the transmission of herpes simplex virus type 2 from men to women. *J Am Med Assoc* 2001; **285**: 3100–3106.

Workowski KA, Berman SM. Sexually transmitted diseases treatment guidelines, 2010. Centers for Disease Control and Prevention. www.cdc.gov/std/treatment/2010, accessed 8/30/2011.

Syphilis Infection in Women

Katherine M. Holman[1] and Alice Goepfert[2]

[1]Department of Medicine, Division of Infectious Diseases, University of Alabama at Birmingham, Birmingham, AL, USA
[2]Department of Obstetrics and Gynecology, Division of Maternal-Fetal Medicine, University of Alabama at Birmingham, Birmingham, AL, USA

Epidemiology

Syphilis remains ever present in modern society. Although reported rates declined in the late 1990s to a low of 2.2 cases/100,000 persons, the last decade has seen a steady increase. The largest increase has been seen in men; however, women have shown a smaller, but no less important, change from 0.8 cases in 2004 to 1.4 cases/100,000 females in 2009, with a disproportionate impact in African-American women living in the southeastern US, as noted in CDC surveillance reports. Rates remain highest in women of younger ages, with 20–24 year olds representing the highest rate of cases in 2009. Factors associated with increased syphilis risk include multiple sexual partners, inconsistent condom use, and partner characteristics.

Clinical presentation

Syphilis is caused by infection with the bacteria, *Treponema pallidum*. It has been called the "great imitator" in reference to its ability to cause a wide range of manifestations in nearly every organ system. Without a high index of suspicion, cases can easily be misdiagnosed. Classically, untreated syphilis progresses through four characteristic stages: primary, secondary, latent, and tertiary.

Primary syphilis

Approximately 1 week to 3 months post exposure to an infected partner, the initial lesion, a chancre (see Figure 5.1) appears. Chancres classically have indurated, symmetric borders, are nontender, and are most often solitary. Importantly, they may occur at any site of exposure – perineum, vagina, cervix, oropharynx, and rectum. Consequently, given the absence of symptoms and the possibility of infection occurring at sites of exposure that can be difficult to visualize, it is relatively common for signs of initial infection – i.e. a vaginal or cervical chancre – to go unnoticed by women. As a result, women are more commonly diagnosed during the secondary stage. Even without appropriate treatment, chancres will spontaneously resolve over a period of a few weeks.

★ TIPS & TRICKS

Primary syphilis usually presents with a chancre. Given its relative lack of symptoms and the possibility of appearance in difficult to visualize places, chancres and consequently primary syphilis are often missed by both provider and patient. As the symptoms spontaneously regress without therapy,

---

Sexually Transmitted Diseases, First Edition. Edited by Richard H. Beigi.
© 2012 John Wiley & Sons, Ltd. Published 2012 by John Wiley & Sons, Ltd.

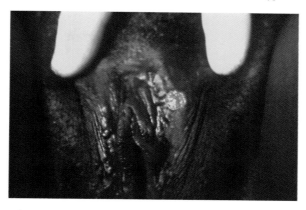

Figure 5.1. Vulvar chancre in patient diagnosed with primary syphilis. (Courtesy of CDC.)

women are commonly not diagnosed until later stages, usually by screening.

This stage represents a time of peak bacteremia and dissemination.

Secondary syphilis

> ★ **TIPS & TRICKS**
>
> Without treatment, concurrent with – or some weeks after – the appearance of the primary chancre, manifestations of secondary syphilis occur in most patients.

Although a range of manifestations is possible (including unnoticed signs), three classic signs will be discussed here: rash, condylomata lata, and mucous patches. Rash most commonly presents in a diffuse maculopapular pattern, often involving the palms and soles (Figure 5.2).

However, the rash may be extremely variable, and can mimic other cutaneous processes, such

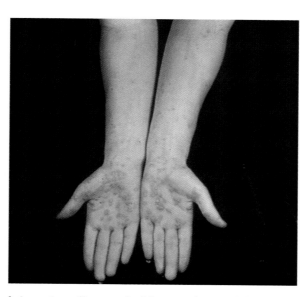

Figure 5.2. Palmer rash in patient diagnosed with secondary syphilis. (Courtesy of CDC/Robert Sumpter.)

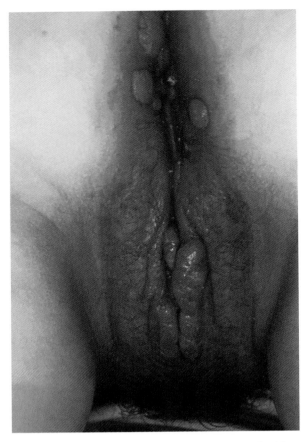

Figure 5.3. Condylomata lata in perineal region of patient diagnosed with secondary syphilis. (Courtesy of CDC/Robert Sumpter.)

as psoriasis, erythema multiforme, pityriasis rosea, or a drug rash. Condylomata lata are moist, raised lesions which usually occur on the upper thighs, labia, or buttocks (Figure 5.3). The lesions can be mistaken for warts; however, condylomata lata typically appear over a period of days to weeks, unlike warts, which grow more slowly. Mucous patches usually occur in the nasolabial folds or oral cavity and resemble silvery-gray patches with surrounding erythema. All these lesions can transmit syphilis, but mucous patches and condylomata lata contain very high concentrations of *T. pallidum* and, consequently, are extremely contagious.

Latent syphilis

Even without therapy, signs from the earlier stages resolve, and untreated patients usually will enter the latent stage, defined as having reactive serologic tests without apparent signs or symptoms. Based on relapse potential and possible infectivity, the latent stage is divided into early ($\leq$ 1 year post-exposure) and late ($\geq$ 1 year post-exposure). Recurrent secondary symptoms occur in approximately 25% of patients during the latent stage. The division of the latent stage into early and late has important implications for both treatment and partner notification guidelines (see below).

Tertiary syphilis

If the infection goes untreated, generally three outcomes are seen: spontaneous resolution of infection, continued latency, or progression to tertiary stage after a period of years to decades. Generally, tertiary manifestations occur as neurosyphilis, cardiovascular syphilis, or gummatous syphilis. All are relatively rare in the USA at the present time.

Diagnosis

As syphilis cannot be cultured with basic laboratory methods, serologic testing is the mainstay of diagnosis. Darkfield microscopy, where available, can be used to evaluate exudate from active lesions, but it remains useful only for positive identification, as three separate samples are required for a definite negative. Serologic diagnosis relies on two different types of test: treponemal, which test for specific treponemal antigens, and nontreponemal, which makes use of cardiolipin–lecithin–cholesterol antigen reactions with antibodies to *T. pallidum*. In the past, a nontreponemal test (RPR, VDRL) was used as the initial/screening test, which, if positive, was then confirmed by a treponemal test (TP-PA, FTA-Ab). The confirmatory testing method is used because nontreponemal tests can have false-positive results due to other etiologies (pregnancy, certain viral infections, rheumatologic diseases, intravenous drug use, etc.). Treponemal tests generally stay positive for life and cannot be used to differentiate between an active or previously treated infection.

More recently, treponemal enzyme and chemiluminescence assays (EIA/CIAs) have been used for the initial screening test in some settings, followed by a nontreponemal test for confirmation. This "reverse sequence" screening has become more common as the EIA is automatable and simpler to use. However, this can lead to discordant test results in which the treponemal test (EIA/CIA) is positive, but the nontreponemal test (RPR, VDRL) is negative. Three such situations could result in a discordant test (1) previous syphilis, with or without prior treatment; (2) very early primary syphilis – nontreponemal antibodies have not yet developed; or (3) a false-positive treponemal test. Given their relative novelty, the Centers for Disease Control and Prevention (CDC) evaluated their use from 2006 to 2010. Findings indicated that discordant results occur more frequently in areas of low prevalence. While the CDC recommends the continued use of traditional screening, if reverse sequence is used and discordant results are found (i.e. +EIA/CIA, –RPR/VDRL), the CDC recommends additional testing with a different treponemal test (TP-PA, FTA-Abs). If this third test is negative, syphilis is unlikely.

A detailed history and physical, including a thorough sexual history, is necessary to evaluate the stage of syphilis, any history of treatment, and any concurrent infections. Any person testing positive for syphilis, should also be tested for HIV as they are common co-infections. Routine screening of asymptomatic individuals in the general population is not recommended. However, routine syphilis screening is recommended in populations considered to be high risk, for example, men who have sex with men, commercial sex workers, persons who exchange sex for drugs, and those with high-risk partners. Optimal intervals for screening in these groups have not been determined. Syphilis screening is also recommended as part of routine prenatal care for all pregnant women due to the potentially devastating consequences of syphilis during pregnancy.

Treatment

Parenteral penicillin remains the standard syphilis treatment, based on more than 50 years of clinical experience. Intramuscular benzathine penicillin is the preparation used in the United States. Treatment is based on the stage at diagnosis in all patients (Table 5.1).

At the time of treatment, all patients should be counseled about the possibility of the Jarisch–Herxheimer reaction, a systemic inflammatory reaction of unknown etiology that can occur around 24–48 hours post-treatment with penicillin. Classically, it presents with fevers, chills, myalgias, headache, and other systemic inflammatory response syndrome criteria. Notably, this does not represent an allergic reaction to penicillin. The reaction generally self-resolves and can be symptomatically treated with fluids and anti-inflammatories. Prednisone, while also effective, is not recommended.

SCIENCE REVISITED

The Jarisch–Herxheimer reaction can occur in 10–25% of patients treated for syphilis. It is characterized by fevers, chills, myalgias, headache, and other systemic inflammatory response syndrome criteria. It represents a systemic inflammatory reaction, although the exact etiology remains unknown. Notably, this does not represent a reaction/allergy to penicillin – a common concern given the possible similarity in symptoms.

Response to therapy

Follow-up to document treatment outcome is imperative – the minimum suggestion is repeating the nontreponemal test used for diagnosis (RPR or VDRL) at 6 and 12 months. Certain clinical situations may warrant more frequent serologic follow-up. Generally, a sustained four-fold decrease in the titer (i.e. 1:16 → 1:4) or seroreversion to negative should be present by 12 months. However, about 15% of patients with early syphilis do not reach the four-fold or 2 dilution decline used to define response to therapy. These patients are referred to as "serofast," and their appropriate management remains an area of debate. Close follow-up and clinical evaluation for the possible need for retreatment is necessary.

Partner management

Reporting a positive syphilis test result to public health authorities is required by law. This allows both case rate determination and partner tracing and notification, often by specially trained Health Department Disease Investigation Specialists (DISs). Although DIS-based partner notification is not commonly done for all sexually transmitted infections, syphilis and HIV are usually prioritized, whereby patients with a positive test are contacted to identify partners and these partners are contacted for testing and treatment (a process known as provider referral). Providers should be knowledgable regarding their local STI reporting policies. The CDC recommends the following contact periods for partner notification by the stage of syphilis: primary (90 days prior to primary lesion onset); secondary (6.5 months prior to secondary symptom onset); and early latent (1 year prior to start of treatment). Although partner notification is important for all patients with syphilis, it remains essential for pregnant women to prevent possible re-exposure and infection of the unborn child.

Special cases

Syphilis in patients with HIV

Screening, utilizing nontreponemal tests, is recommended at baseline and at least annually in all sexually active persons with HIV. More frequent screening may be indicated on the basis of risk factors. Diagnosis and treatment regimens are the same for syphilis patients with HIV coinfection. However, because of concerns about the possibility of increased treatment failure generated from case reports and small series, closer follow-up is recommended with nontreponemal test titer measurements at 3, 6, 9, 12, and 24 months. While there are some concerns that patients with HIV may have unusual serologic responses, a higher risk for neurosyphilis, and are possibly more likely to experience treatment failure, the CDC does not recommend any changes in the treatment regimen from that recommended for HIV-negative patients.

Syphilis in pregnancy

Screening during pregnancy is the mainstay of prevention for congenital syphilis. Syphilis is a particularly important disease to evaluate for, given its long clinical latency, the availability of effective therapy, and the potentially devastating outcomes if a mother/unborn child are not treated appropriately. Rates of vertical transmission are reported as 70–100% in primary syphilis cases, and 40% in early latent cases.

Screening/treatment

All pregnant women should be screened at their first prenatal visit utilizing the same protocol as for nonpregnant patients, and those at high risk (i.e. living in area with a high incidence of syphilis, multiple sex partners, or no previous documented screening) should be rescreened at approximately 28 weeks and again at delivery. Any pregnant woman who is a known sexual contact to a person diagnosed with syphilis, should be treated empirically. As local laws or health department guidelines may be more stringent and supersede these recommendations, providers should be familiar with their local policies. Complete treatment of syphilis in pregnant women ideally should occur ≥30 days before delivery, utilizing the penicillin regimen

Table 5.1. Recommended regimens for nonpregnant patients (adapted from 2010 CDC STD Treatment Guidelines)

Stage	Recommended	Alternative for penicillin allergic
Primary/secondary	2.4 million units benzathine penicillin IM × 1	Doxycycline 100 mg po BID × 14 days
Early latent	2.4 million units benzathine penicillin IM × 1	Doxycycline 100 mg po BID × 14 days
Late latent or unknown duration	2.4 million units benzathine penicillin IM × 3 doses, given over 3 weeks at 1 week intervals	Doxycycline 100 mg po BID × 28 days
Tertiary without evidence of neurosyphilis	2.4 million units benzathine penicillin IM × 3 doses, given over 3 weeks at 1 week intervals	Consult with specialist
Neurosyphilis	Aqueous crystalline penicillin G 18–24 million units per day, administered as 3–4 million units IV every 4 hours or continuous infusion, for 10–14 days	Consult with specialist

appropriate for the patient's stage of syphilis. The CDC states that no change in the treatment of syphilis is required for pregnant women. However, patients with penicillin allergies need to be desensitized in the hospital, and then treated immediately after desensitization. No alternatives to penicillin are recommended for therapy in pregnant women (Table 5.2). If available, allergy testing may be performed to confirm penicillin allergy; if the full battery is negative, the patient can be treated without desensitization. An excellent overview of allergy testing recommendations is available in the most recent CDC STD Treatment Guidelines. Erythromycin has not been shown to reliably cure an infected fetus; tetracyclines should be avoided due to fetal toxicity.

For women diagnosed during the second half of pregnancy, two concerns arise: (1) need for ultrasound evaluation of the fetus and (2) concern for premature labor and/or fetal distress if the patient experiences the Jarisch–Herxheimer reaction. The CDC now recommends ultrasound evaluation of the fetus at the time of syphilis diagnosis for evidence of congenital syphilis as this may indicate an increased risk of fetal treatment failure. Following treatment, women in the second half of their pregnancy should be counseled to seek immediate obstetric care if they experience fever, contractions, or a decrease in fetal movement. However, concern over either of these possibilities should not delay maternal therapy for diagnosed syphilis.

Some experts have recommended an increased number/dosage of benzathine PCN in the treatment of a pregnant woman with syphilis. This concern arises from cohort studies evaluating failure/success rates of both the CDC guidelines as well as increased PCN regimens. Donders et al. (1997) investigated a planned regimen of 7.2 million units of benzathine PCN over 3 weeks, which did not show a significant decrease in congenital syphilis, but patients who received 2 or 3 injections showed lower rates of prematurity and neonatal mortality. Notably, most of the women who did not complete treatment delivered less than 4 weeks from any PCN injection. Alexander et al. (1999) examined an additional large cohort involving patients with early (primary, secondary, early latent) and late latent syphilis, evaluating the CDC recommended treatment

Table 5.2. Recommended regimens for pregnant patients (adapted from 2010 CDC STD Treatment Guidelines)

Stage	Recommended	Alternative for penicillin allergic
Primary/secondary	2.4 million units benzathine penicillin IM × 1	Consult with specialist
Early latent	2.4 million units benzathine penicillin IM × 1	Consult with specialist
Late latent or unknown duration	2.4 million units benzathine penicillin IM × 3 doses, given over 3 weeks at 1 week intervals	Consult with specialist
Tertiary without evidence of neurosyphilis	2.4 million units benzathine penicillin IM × 3 doses, given over 3 weeks at 1 week intervals	Consult with specialist
Neurosyphilis	Aqueous crystalline penicillin G 18–24 million units per day, administered as 3–4 million units IV every 4 hours or continuous infusion, for 10–14 days	Consult with specialist

guidelines, which demonstrated an efficacy of 98.2%, with the only significant decrease in success rate seen in secondary syphilis.

Follow-up post-treatment should include the measurement of titers in the third trimester and at delivery. Although monthly titers have been recommended in the past, fetal treatment failure does not seem to be predicted by maternal serologic response. However, monthly titers may still be considered in patients at high risk of reinfection, i.e. those who live in high prevalence areas. Appropriate response to therapy (i.e. a four-fold decline in titer) ideally should be documented 30 days prior to delivery. If this has not/cannot be done at the time of delivery, the evaluation of the neonate should be based on the recommendations in the most recent CDC STD treatment guidelines. No child born to a mother with serologic evidence of and/or no documented evaluation for syphilis during the pregnancy should leave the hospital prior to evaluation and possible treatment.

Congenital syphilis

The most recent CDC data from 2009 reported a rate of 10.0 cases/100,000 live births in the United States. The stage of syphilis present during pregnancy may have an effect on fetal outcome –

infants born to women with primary or secondary syphilis are more likely to be born prematurely, or have perinatal death, than those born to women with latent infection. Late or limited prenatal care remains a risk for congenital syphilis, but nonadherence to screening guidelines also contributes.

⚖ SCIENCE REVISITED

Overall, the rate of congenital syphilis has been increasing since 2005, concurrently with an increase in the rates of primary and secondary syphilis in women since 2004. Given this temporal relationship, an increased risk for congenital syphilis is seen in the same groups that are at high risk for primary and secondary syphilis.

Case definition of congenital syphilis

Surveillance: Created by CDC to provide rapid case surveillance (ideally used shortly after birth) and to provide a simpler classification with standardization to allow for comparison across regions.

Clinical: Signs in infants <2 years old include snuffles, condylomata lata (both highly contagious), rash, hepatosplenomegaly, jaundice, edema, anemia, or pseudoparalysis. Stigmata in older children include mulberry molars, Hutchinson teeth, saddle nose, anterior bowing of shins, frontal bossing, nerve deafness, interstitial keratitis, rhagades or Clutton joints.

As only the most severe cases will be evident at birth (or as syphilitic stillbirths), diagnosis can be difficult. The surveillance definition, as it is used at a single time point, may result in over inclusion and thus, overtreatment. However, given the potentially devastating outcomes of untreated syphilis in a neonate, compared to the relatively low risk of therapy (i.e. penicillin), overtreatment is preferred.

Summary

Syphilis remains a disease of considerable public health importance. Variable clinical presentations make screening essential in high-risk groups, as well as in pregnant women. Diagnosis relies on a detailed clinical and physical examination, along with serological testing. Treatment is based on the stage at diagnosis. Penicillin is the mainstay of therapy, and is the only acceptable option for pregnant women diagnosed with syphilis. Follow-up with sequential serologic testing to document appropriate response to treatment is particularly important in pregnant women, preferably documenting response 30 days before delivery. Any baby born to a woman without any screening or who doesnot have documented treatment and appropriate response needs to be evaluated for signs/symptoms of congenital syphilis, and considered for penicillin therapy prior to discharge. Early diagnosis and intervention are necessary to decrease the morbidity from syphilis.

Bibliography

Aberg JA, Kaplan JE, Libman H, et al. Primary care guidelines for the management of persons infected with human immunodeficiency virus: 2009 update by the HIV Medicine Association of the Infectious Diseases Society of America. *Clin Infect Dis* 2009; **49**: 651–681.

Alexander JM, Sheffield JS, Sanchez PJ, et al. Efficacy of treatment for syphilis in pregnancy. *Obstet Gynecol* 1999; **93**: 5–8.

American Academy of Pediatrics Committee on Fetus and Newborn and the American College of Obstetricians and Gynecologists Committee on Obstetrics. Perinatal infections. In: *Guidelines for Perinatal Care*, 6th edn. AAP (Grove Park, IL) and ACOG (Washington, DC), 2007; pp. 303–348.

Augenbraun M. Syphilis. In: *Current Diagnosis & Treatment: Sexually Transmitted Diseases* (Klausner JD, Hook EW III, eds.). McGraw-Hill Medical: New York, NY, 2007; pp. 119–129.

Centers for Disease Control and Prevention. *Sexually Transmitted Disease Surveillance 2000 Syphilis Surveillance Report.* Division of STD Prevention, US Department of Health and Human Services: Atlanta, December 2001.

Centers for Disease Control and Prevention. Congenital syphilis case investigation and reporting form instructions. Form: CDC 73.126 REV. 10-2003. http://www.cdc.gov/std/program/ConSyphInstr11-2003.pdf. Accessed March 31, 2011.

Centers for Disease Control and Prevention. Discordant results from reverse sequence syphilis screening – five laboratories, United States, 2006–2010. *MMWR* 2011 Feb; **60**(5): 133–137.

Centers for Disease Control and Prevention. Primary and secondary syphilis – Jefferson County, Alabama, 2002–2007. *MMWR* 2009 May 8; **58** (17):463–467.

Centers for Disease Control and Prevention. *Sexually Transmitted Disease Surveillance 2009.* US Department of Health and Human Services: Atlanta, 2010.

Centers for Disease Control and Prevention. Sexually transmitted diseases treatment guidelines, 2010. *MMWR* 2010; **59** (No. RR-12): 1–110.

Centers for Disease Control and Prevention. Sexually transmitted diseases treatment guidelines. *MMWR* 1993; **42** (No. RR-14).

Donders GG, Desmyter J, Hooft P, Dewet GH. Apparent failure of one injection of benzathine penicillin G for syphilis during pregnancy in human immunodeficiency virus-seronegative African women. *Sex Transm Dis* 1997; **24**: 94–101.

Doroshenko A, Sherrard J, Pollard AJ. Syphilis in pregnancy and the neonatal period. *Internat Journal STD & AIDS* 2006; **17**: 221–228.

Golden MR, Faxelid E, Low N. Partner notification for sexually transmitted infections including HIV infection: an evidence-based assessment. In: *Sexually Transmitted Diseases*, 4th edn. (Holmes K, et al., eds.). McGraw-Hill Medical: New York, NY, 2008; pp. 965–984.

Hitti J, Watts DH. Bacterial sexually transmitted infections in pregnancy. In: *Sexually Transmitted Diseases*, 4th edn. (Holmes K, et al., eds.). McGraw-Hill Medical: New York, NY, 2008; pp. 1529–1561.

Larsen SA, Steiner BM, Rudolph AH. Laboratory diagnosis and interpretation of tests for syphilis. *Clin Microbiol Rev* 1995; **8**: 1–21.

Sparling PF, Swartz MN, Musher DM, Healy BP. Clinical manifestations of syphilis. In: *Sexually Transmitted Diseases*, 4th edn. (Holmes K, et al., eds.). McGraw-Hill Medical: New York, NY, 2008; pp. 661–684.

Tramont EC. *Treponema pallidum* (Syphilis). In: *Mandell, Douglas, and Bennett's: Principles and Practice of Infectious Diseases*, Vol II, 7th edn. (Mandell GL, et al., eds.). Elsevier: Philadelphia, PA, 2010; pp. 3035–3053.

US Preventative Services Task Force. Screening for syphilis infection: recommendation statement. *Ann Fam Med* 2004; **2**: 362–365.

Wendel GD, Sheffield JS, Hollier LM, et al. Treatment of syphilis in pregnancy and prevention of congenital syphilis. *Clin Infect Dis* 2002; **35** (Suppl 2): S200–S209.

Chancroid and Lymphogranuloma Venereum

Tracy L. Lemonovich and Robert A. Salata

Division of Infectious Disease and HIV Medicine, University Hospitals Case Medical Center, Case Western Reserve University, Cleveland, OH, USA

Chancroid (Haemophilus ducreyi)

Introduction

Haemophilus ducreyi is the causative agent of chancroid, an infection characterized by genital ulcers and inguinal lymphadenitis. Although relatively uncommon in the United States, it is a significant cause of genital ulcer disease in resource-limited settings (RLS), particularly sub-Saharan Africa. Definitive diagnosis of chancroid is challenging, likely underestimating its overall prevalence.

Microbiologic etiology and pathogenesis

H. ducreyi is a small, highly fastidious, Gram-negative coccobacillus which has a hemin nutritional requirement necessitating selective medium for growth. *H. ducreyi* was classified as a *Haemophilus* species due to its biochemical properties, growth requirements, and related antigens to other species in this group. However, *H. ducreyi* has more recently been shown by rRNA analysis to be only distantly related to other haemophili such as *H. influenzae*. *H. ducreyi* is now classified in the Pasteurellaceae family. *H. ducreyi* is strictly a human pathogen without any animal or environmental reservoirs. Infection occurs through inoculation of the bacteria via breaks in the epithelium during sexual contact with an infected individual. The bacterium is highly infectious, with a human experimental model demonstrating papule formation in 50% of cases with an inoculation of a single colony forming unit (cfu). Upon infection, the bacteria remain extracellular and co-localize with polymorphonuclear leukocytes (PMNs), macrophages, collagen, and fibrin. Evasion of phagocytosis and phagocytic killing appear to be an important immune evasion mechanism in the pathogenesis of infection. Several bacterial virulence factors have been identified, including lipo-oligosaccarides (LOS), pili, heat shock proteins, outer membrane proteins, and cytotoxins. *H. ducreyi* secretes a cytolethal distending toxin (CDT) which may play an important role in the development or persistence of ulcerative lesions via epithelial cell injury. Ulcerative lesions of chancroid are associated with a mononuclear cell infiltrate in the dermis, consisting of significant numbers of CD4+ T lymphocytes. This cutaneous infiltrate of CD4+ T cells provides a mechanism which can facilitate human immunodeficiency virus (HIV) transmission by *H. ducreyi*. Natural infection does not confer protective immunity; hence patients may become reinfected with chancroid. This has also been demonstrated in experimental human models of infection with *H. ducreyi*.

Epidemiology

In the United States, chancroid cases reported to the Centers for Disease Control and Prevention

Sexually Transmitted Diseases, First Edition. Edited by Richard H. Beigi.

© 2012 John Wiley & Sons, Ltd. Published 2012 by John Wiley & Sons, Ltd.

(CDC) declined steadily from the 1980s until the early 2000s. Since that time, the number of cases annually have fluctuated but remained relatively low. Most cases of chancroid in the USA are reported from eastern cities and the south. In the most recent reported surveillance data from 2009, only 28 cases were reported from nine states. Although this likely represents an overall decline in the incidence of disease, difficulty in diagnosis and lack of awareness make underdiagnosis a concern. This is illustrated by several studies demonstrating that a significant number of genital ulcers in the USA are caused by *H. ducreyi* when this etiology is tested for. Chancroid is also a significant cause of outbreaks of genital ulcer disease, and is epidemiologically linked to increased HIV seroprevalence. *H. ducreyi* was the cause of an outbreak of genital ulcer disease in Jackson, Mississippi, in 1994 in 39% of cases tested by a multiplex polymerase chain reaction (PCR) assay. When evaluated in the context of outbreaks, chancroid is more commonly reported among minority populations, particularly African-Americans and Hispanics. Chancroid cases are also more frequently reported in men than in women, which is at least partly explained by the disease being more easily diagnosed in men. Transmission primarily occurs in heterosexuals, and there is a strong association between chancroid and illicit drug use, commercial sex workers, and exchange of sex for drugs.

In RLS, chancroid is a major cause of genital ulcer disease in sub-Saharan Africa, Latin America, and Southeast Asia. However, the true prevalence of chancroid is unknown in many of these endemic areas due to limited resources available for diagnosis. As in the USA, several studies of developing countries have noted recent decreases in cases of genital ulcer disease secondary to *H. ducreyi*, with a subsequent increase in proportion of genital ulcer disease due to herpes simplex virus (HSV). This decrease in chancroid prevalence in RLS countries may be due to increase in regular sexually transmitted infection (STI) screening and empiric antibiotic therapy for genital ulcer disease.

Clinical manifestations

The incubation period for *H. ducreyi* infection is usually 2–5 days from inoculation to the development of symptoms. The classic manifestation of chancroid is genital ulceration. The infection commonly begins as a papule, which then promptly evolves into a pustule before eroding into a deep, undermined, purulent ulcer. Typical ulcers are painful, non-indurated, well circumscribed with ragged edges, and often with gray or yellow necrotic material at the base. Multiple ulcers may occur and can coalesce into a large area of ulceration. Approximately half of patients have regional inguinal lymphadenopathy with bubo formation, which may become fluctuant and rupture spontaneously (Figure 6.1). Ulceration may resolve spontaneously prior to the development of adenopathy and suppuration. The most common sites of ulceration include the glans penis, corona, or prepuce in men and the labia or vaginal introitus in women. *H. ducreyi* does not systemically disseminate but extragenital lesions rarely occur, likely due to autoinoculation. Untreated ulcers may persist for 1–3 months without treatment. The presence of concomitant HIV infection may lead to an atypical presentation of chancroid, such as multiple ulcers, longer duration of ulceration, and extragenital lesions.

The differential diagnosis of chancroid is broad, and consists of other causes of genital ulcer disease, including primary syphilis with a chancre, genital herpes, lymphogranuloma venereum, and donovanosis. More than one pathogen may also be present in a single patient, particularly coinfection between chancroid and primary syphilis. In the USA the most common cause of genital ulcer disease is HSV, followed by syphilis and chancroid. Noninfectious causes of genital ulcer disease also should be considered, including a fixed drug eruption and Behçet syndrome.

Diagnosis

The diagnosis of chancroid is difficult due to the lack of availability of diagnostic testing in most laboratories, even in industrialized nations. Given these limitations, a clinical diagnosis of chancroid is commonly used, although this has been shown to be often insensitive and/or nonspecific. The CDC has defined clinical criteria for a probable diagnosis of chancroid as a guide for surveillance and initiation of therapy. The

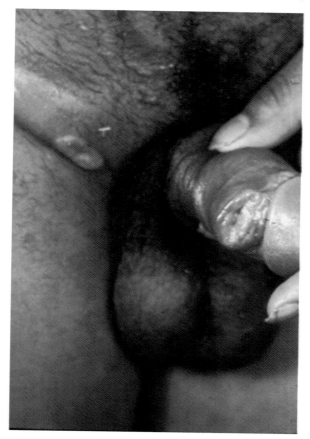

Figure 6.1. Chancroid penile lesion and inguinal lymphadenopathy. (Courtesy of Centers for Disease Control and Prevention, Division of STD Prevention, STD Clinical Slides.)

probable diagnosis can be made if all the following criteria are met: (1) the patient has one or more painful genital ulcers; (2) the patient has no evidence of *T. pallidum* infection by darkfield examination of ulcer exudate or by a serologic test for syphilis performed at least 7 days after the onset of ulcers; (3) the clinical presentation, appearance of genital ulcers and, if present, regional lymphadenopathy are typical for chancroid; and (4) a test for HSV performed on the ulcer exudate is negative.

A definitive diagnosis of chancroid requires the laboratory isolation of *H. ducreyi* and should be sought for confirmation of the diagnosis whenever possible. Gram stain of ulcer exudate can reveal small Gram-negative coccobacilli in chains (Figure 6.2) or with a classic "school of fish"

pattern, but sensitivity is less than 50%. The identification of *H. ducreyi* from culture of ulcer exudate or aspirate of suppurative lymphadenopathy confirms the diagnosis, but the organism is difficult to grow and requires selective media that is not widely available. Developments in culture media have improved the yield, with the reported sensitivity of culture being approximately 75%. Nonculture methods for detection of *H. ducreyi*, specifically PCR, are the most promising approach for diagnosis. Multiplex PCR for *H. ducreyi* has been associated with sensitivities of greater than 95% in several studies. There is no FDA-approved PCR test for *H. ducreyi* in the USA, but testing can be done by commercial laboratories that have developed and verified their own test. Unfortunately, these tests are not readily

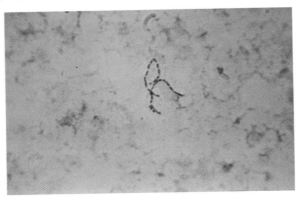

Figure 6.2. Gram stain *H. ducreyi*. (Courtesy of Centers for Disease Control and Prevention, Division of STD Prevention, STD Clinical Slides.)

available to most sexually transmitted disease (STD) clinics and, when done, results are not immediately known, therefore treatment decisions are not usually able to be made on the basis of microbiologic testing. Serologic antibody testing has been used to evaluate the prevalence of chancroid epidemiologically, but is not clinically useful in determining an acute cause of genital ulcer disease.

Treatment

Empiric therapy for a suspected diagnosis of chancroid should be considered on the basis of a typical clinical presentation with supportive epidemiology while laboratory studies are pending. The successful treatment of chancroid involves cure of the infection, resolution of clinical symptoms, and prevention of transmission to sexual contacts. A number of antibiotic agents have been used in the treatment of chancroid; single-dose directly observed therapy is desirable to ensure that the appropriate therapy is completed. The CDC recommended regimens for treatment include single-dose azithromycin 1 g orally or ceftriaxone 250 mg intramuscularly. Azithromycin treatment has been associated with cure rates of approximately 90%, with ceftriaxone treatment cure rates as high as 98%. Alternative regimens include ciprofloxacin 500 mg orally twice daily for 3 days and erythromycin base 500 mg orally three times daily for 7 days, but these regimens have the disadvantage of requir-

ing multiple doses over several days that may be associated with nonadherence. Ceftriaxone is the treatment of choice in pregnancy. Resistant *H. ducreyi* isolates have been reported to antimicrobial agents that were previously effective, such as widespread resistance to trimethoprim-sulfamethoxazole. Rare quinolone resistance has also been reported.

Clinical improvement usually occurs quickly after the start of therapy, with symptomatic pain relief within 3 days and objective improvement in ulcers within 7 days. Uncircumcised men and patients infected with HIV may not respond as promptly to therapy. Patients should be evaluated within 3 to 7 days after initiation of treatment. If clinical response does not occur within 7 days, consideration should be made regarding a possible incorrect diagnosis, coinfection with another STD (especially syphilis), coinfection with HIV, treatment nonadherence, or *H. ducreyi* drug-resistance. All patients treated for chancroid should be tested for syphilis and HIV, with repeat testing at 3 months if initial testing is negative. The sex partners of patients with chancroid should be evaluated and treated for chancroid if they had sexual contact with the patient within 10 days of onset of symptoms, even if the contact is asymptomatic. Fluctuant lymphadenitis should be treated with needle aspiration or incision and drainage to prevent the development of draining fistulas or secondary ulcers. In advanced cases, scarring can occur even with successful therapy.

Lymphogranuloma venereum

(*Chlamydia trachomatis* serovars L1, L2, L3)

Introduction

Lymphogranuloma venereum (LGV) is caused by *Chlamydia trachomatis* serovars L1, L2, and L3, and is characterized by genital ulcerations and lymphadenopathy. LGV is endemic to tropical and subtropical regions of the world, and causes sporadic disease in the developed world. Diagnosis is difficult to make solely on clinical symptoms, and requires a high degree of suspicion as well as additional laboratory studies for confirmation.

Microbiologic etiology and pathogenesis

C. trachomatis is one of four species within the family Chlamydiaceae, which are nonmotile obligate intracellular prokaryotic organisms with a unique biphasic life cycle. The elementary body is the extracellular transmissible form of the organism that attaches to a susceptible epithelial cell to initiate the life cycle. *C. trachomatis* can then enter the cell via phagocytosis, pinocytosis, or receptor-mediated endocytosis, although these mechanisms have not been fully elucidated. The reticulate body is the intracellular form of the organism, and replicates within the host cell. The chlamydiae then exit the host cell at the end of the growth cycle by either lysis or extrusion. The life cycle of the organism takes between 48 and 72 hours. The LGV serovars of *C. trachomatis* enter the body through the genital or rectal mucosal epithelial cells or breaks in the skin, and then migrate to regional lymph nodes via lymphatic drainage. Systemic dissemination with bacteremia can occur. Chlamydiae appear to induce tissue inflammation and damage via induction of cytokines such as interleukin-8 (IL-8). The endotoxin lipopolysaccharide may be the main chlamydial antigen that induces these pro-inflammatory cytokines. Data suggests that *C. trachomatis* is also able to downregulate aspects of the host immune response to promote long-lasting infection. Natural infection with *C. trachomatis* confers limited protection against reinfection, although both cell-mediated and antibody-mediated mechanisms have been identified that confer partial, often short-term, immunity.

Epidemiology

LGV is known to be endemic in Africa, India, Southeast Asia, South America, and the Caribbean. Despite a high frequency of seropositivity to *C. trachomatis*, LGV causes a relatively low overall proportion of genital ulcer disease in these regions compared to other etiologies such as HSV, syphilis, or chancroid. However, the true prevalence of LGV is difficult to determine in RLS due to limitations in diagnostic capabilities.

Although relatively rare in industrialized countries, LGV has become an increasingly important cause of outbreaks of proctitis in North America, the United Kingdom, and Europe in the last 10 years, particularly in men who have sex with men (MSM). A previously undescribed *C. trachomatis* serovar, L2b, was identified as the main causative serovar in this epidemic, suggesting a close epidemiological link among the outbreaks. There has been a strong association between LGV and HIV infection in the MSM population, with HIV prevalence among LGV cases ranging from 67% to 100% in a meta-analysis of 13 studies. Other risk factors for LGV in MSM include coinfection with hepatitis C virus, diagnosis of other sexually transmitted infections, and high-risk sexual practices such as unprotected anal intercourse, multiple sex partners, and use of the internet and sex-on-premises venues for meeting sex partners. There is still significant debate regarding the role of the asymptomatic carriage of *C. trachomatis* LGV serovars as a source of LGV infection in MSM, with conflicting data on the prevalence of subclinical infection.

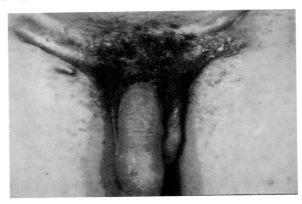

Figure 6.3. Lymphogranuloma venereum inguinal lymphadenopathy. (Courtesy of Centers for Disease Control and Prevention, Division of STD Prevention, STD Clinical Slides.)

Clinical manifestations

The classic presentation of LGV occurs in three distinct stages. Primary infection is characterized by the development of a primary lesion at the site of inoculation, usually a small papule, ulcer, or mucosal inflammatory reaction. The most common sites for primary lesions are the prepuce or glans penis in men and the vulva, vaginal wall, or cervix in women. Other potential sites of primary infection include the urethra and rectum. The incubation period for infection is between 3 and 30 days. The primary lesion is typically painless and self-limited, usually healing within a few days without scarring. It is often unrecognized by the patient until the secondary stage develops. The secondary stage of infection occurs days to weeks after the primary infection, and symptoms are related to the extension of infection to regional lymph nodes, causing lymphadenopathy and often systemic symptoms such as fever, myalgias, and headache. The lymph nodes involved are dependent on the initial site of inoculation, usually inguinal nodes in men with primary penile infection (Figure 6.3), inguinal and femoral nodes in women with primary vulvar infection, and deep iliac nodes with primary rectal infection.

Lymphadenopathy is usually unilateral; the classic "groove sign" is indicated by the presence of adenopathy above and below the inguinal ligament which occurs in approximately 10–20% of LGV cases. The lymphadenopathy may coalesce to form an inflammatory mass or bubo, which may spontaneously rupture and form fistulas or sinus tracts. An anorectal syndrome may also develop which is characterized by proctocolitis and an inflammatory mass in the rectum and retroperitoneum due to proliferation of intestinal and perirectal lymphatic tissue. This syndrome may lead to chronic complications such as colorectal fistulae and strictures. Patients often have systemic symptoms such as fever in addition to anorectal pain, rectal discharge, constipation, and/or tenesmus. The third stage of infection is characterized by chronic inflammation of the genital tract, which may involve fibrosis and lymphatic obstruction leading to genital elephantiasis (Figure 6.4), fistulae, strictures, or infertility.

The differential diagnosis of LGV includes other causes of genital ulcer disease and lymphadenopathy, including primary syphilis, genital herpes, chancroid, and donovanosis. Coinfection of LGV genital or colorectal lesions with other sexually transmitted infections as well as nonsexually transmitted bacterial superinfection may occur.

Diagnosis

The diagnosis of LGV is difficult to establish on a clinical basis alone, and laboratory confirmation of *C. trachomatis* should be pursued when possible. For patients with genital infection, genital or lymph node specimens (lesion swab or bubo aspirate) can be tested for *C. trachomatis* by culture, direct immunofluorescence, or nucleic acid detection. Overall, culture yield is low from genital and lymph node aspirates, with the organism being isolated from bubo purulence by

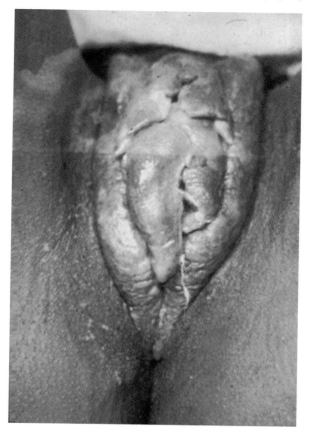

Figure 6.4. Female genital elephantiasis due to lymphogranuloma venereum. (Courtesy of Centers for Disease Control and Prevention, Division of STD Prevention, STD Clinical Slides.)

culture in approximately 30% of cases of LGV, with a lower frequency of isolation from other sites such as the cervix or urethra. Specific chlamydia cultures are also not widely available outside of referral centers. Antigen detection by a direct immunofluorescence (DFA) or enzyme-linked immunosorbent assay (EIA) can be done on ulcer or lymph node aspirate specimens. Antigen detection has several limitations, including the need for significant technical expertise for DFA and the low sensitivity of some EIA tests, and therefore this diagnostic modality has largely been supplanted by nucleic acid amplification testing (NAAT). NAATs detect chlamydial DNA or RNA and are highly sensitive and specific. Additionally, this method can be used to differentiate between LGV and non-LGV serovars by PCR-based genotyping, and can be used on rectal swab specimens in

addition to other sites. Unfortunately, this genotyping technology is still not widely available, but can be done through the CDC via local or state laboratories when appropriate. There is no FDA-approved NAAT for *C. trachomatis* testing of rectal specimens, but some commercial laboratories have validated their own tests for clinical use. Chlamydia serology, by complement fixation (CF) or microimmunofluorescence (MIF), is not diagnostic, but can support the diagnosis of LGV in the appropriate clinical context. Most serologic tests are limited by the inability to distinguish between the *C. trachomatis* serovars, and a serologic test interpretation is not standardized. However, an IgG titer of >1:64 can strengthen the diagnosis of LGV in the correct clinical context, and a titer <1:32 argues against the diagnosis, except very early in the infection. Histopathologic changes are also not specific, but may support the diagnosis. A skin test of delayed hypersensitivity to chlamydial antigens, the Frei test, is of historical interest but is no longer available.

Treatment

The CDC recommended preferred regimen for the treatment of LGV, including proctitis, is doxycycline 100 mg orally twice daily for 21 days. The alternative regimen is erythromycin base 500 mg four times a day for 21 days, which is also the treatment of choice during pregnancy. Treatment with azithromycin 1 g orally weekly for 3 weeks and prolonged fluoroquinolone-based regimens may also be effective. Treatment cures the infection and stops further tissue damage, but scarring may result even with adequate treatment if given late in the course of the infection. The prolonged duration of treatment recommended is based on clinical experience with recurrence using short-course therapy, and is supported by studies showing prolonged shedding of chlamydial RNA of >14 days even after the initiation of appropriate antimicrobial therapy. All patients should be followed for resolution of signs and symptoms of infection, and patients with HIV may have a delay in resolution and/or require more prolonged therapy. Buboes may require needle aspiration or incision and drainage to avoid the development of fistulae or sinus tracts related to rupture. All patients diagnosed with LGV should be tested for HIV. Partners who had sexual contact with a LGV patient within 60 days of the onset of the patient's symptoms should be examined, tested for urethral or cervical chlamydial infection, and treated with a standard chlamydial regimen of azithromycin 1 g orally single dose or doxycycline 100 mg orally twice daily for 7 days.

> ### ⚠ CAUTION!
>
> A prolonged treatment of 21 days with doxycycline is necessary for adequate treatment of LGV. Patients with HIV may have a delay in response or require a more extended course of therapy. Recurrence of infection may occur with shorter-course treatment.

Bibliography

Batteiger BE, Xu F, Johnson RE, et al. Protective immunity to *Chlamydia trachomatis* genital infection: evidence from human studies. *J Infect Dis* 2010; **201** (Suppl 2): S178–S189.

Bong CT, Bauer ME, Spinola SM. *Haemophilus ducreyi*: clinical features, epidemiology, and prospects for disease control. *Microbes Infect* 2002; **4**: 1141–1148.

Centers for Disease Control and Prevention, Division of Sexually Transmitted Diseases. Sexually Transmitted Diseases Surveillance, Other Sexually Transmitted Diseases, 2009 National Report. (http://www.cdc.gov/std/stats09/other.htm). Accessed April 9, 2011.

Chen CY, Chi KH, Alexander S. A real-time quadriplex PCR assay for the diagnosis of rectal lymphogranuloma venereum and non-lymphogranuloma venereum *Chlamydia trachomatis* infections. *Sex Transm Infect* 2008; **84**: 273–276.

de Vries HJ, Smelov V, Middelburg JG, et al. Delayed microbial cure of lymphogranuloma venereum proctitis with doxycycline treatment. *Clin Infect Dis* 2009; **48**: 53–56.

Lewis DA. Chancroid: clinical manifestations, diagnosis, and management. *Sex Transm Infect* 2003; **79**: 68–71.

Mabey D, Peeling RW. Lymphogranuloma venereum. *Sex Transm Infect* 2002; **78**: 90–92.

Martin-Iguacel R, Llibre JM, Nielsen H, et al. Lymphogranuloma venereum proctocolitis: a silent endemic disease in men who have sex with men in industrialised countries. *Eur J Clin Microbiol Infect Dis* 2010; **29**: 917–925.

McLean CA, Stoner BP, Workowski KA. Treatment of lymphogranuloma venereum. *Clin Infect Dis* 2007; **44** (Suppl 3): S147–S152.

Mertz KJ, Trees D, Levine WC, et al. Etiology of genital ulcers and prevalence of human immunodeficiency virus coinfection in 10 US cities. The Genital Ulcer Disease Surveillance Group. *J Infect Dis* 1998; **178**: 1795–1798.

Moulder JW. Interaction of chlamydiae and host cells in vitro. *Microbiol Rev* 1991; **55**: 143–190.

Pathela P, Blank S, Schillinger JA. Lymphogranuloma venereum: old pathogen, new story. *Curr Infect Dis Rep* 2007; **9**: 143–150.

Ronn MM, Ward H. The association between lymphogranuloma venereum and HIV among men who have sex with men: systematic review and meta-analysis. *BMC Infect Dis* 2011; **11**: 70.

Sethi G, Allason-Jones E, Richens J, et al. Lymphogranuloma venereum presenting as genital ulceration and inguinal syndrome in men who have sex with men in London, UK. *Sex Transm Infect* 2009; **85**: 165–170.

Spinola SM, Bauer ME, Munson RS Jr. Immunopathogenesis of Haemophilus ducreyi infection (chancroid). *Infect Immun* 2002; **70**: 1667–1676.

Taylor-Robinson D. Evaluation and comparison of tests to diagnose *Chlamydia trachomatis* genital infections. *Hum Reprod* 1997; **12**: 113–120.

Trees DL, Morse SA. Chancroid and *Haemophilus ducreyi*: an update. *Clin Microbiol Rev* 1995; **8**: 357–375.

Ward H, Alexander S, Carder C, et al. The prevalence of lymphogranuloma venereum infection in men who have sex with men: results of a multicentre case finding study. *Sex Transm Infect* 2009; **85**: 173–175.

Ward H, Martin I, Macdonald N, et al. Lymphogranuloma venereum in the United Kingdom. *Clin Infect Dis* 2007; **44**: 26–32.

Workowski KA, Berman S, Centers for Disease Control and Prevention (CDC). Sexually transmitted diseases treatment guidelines, 2010. *MMWR Recomm Rep* 2010; **59**: 1–110.

Bacterial Vaginosis

Jeanne M. Marrazzo

Division of Allergy and Infectious Diseases, University of Washington, and Division of Infectious Diseases, Harborview Medical Center, Seattle, WA, USA

Introduction

Bacterial vaginosis (BV) is the most prevalent form of vaginal infection in women of reproductive age, affecting 8% to 23%, and is the most common etiology of vaginal symptoms prompting women to seek medical care. BV represents a condition in which the normal protective lactobacilli are replaced by high quantities of commensal anaerobes, resulting in symptomatic vaginitis in many women. Symptomatic BV, which accounts for approximately 60% of all cases, typically causes abnormal vaginal discharge that is increased in amount, typically gray and uniformly adherent to the vaginal mucosa (Figure 7.1) and often malodorous. The odor, usually described as "fishy," is derived from volatilization of the amines that result from the metabolism of the copious anaerobic bacteria that characterize this disorder. In clinical practice, the evaluation of women with BV – or, for that matter, of women with any vaginal complaint — is often complicated by the fact that over-the-counter antifungal vaginal medications are frequently used for the self-treatment of vaginal symptoms that are actually due to BV.

Globally, BV is very common. Of 3,739 women enrolled during 2001–2004 in a nationally representative sample of the US civilian noninstitutionalized population, almost one in three (29.2%; 95% CI: 27.2–31.3) had BV by Gram stain of vaginal fluid. In that study, women were more likely to have BV if they were nonwhite or reported douching, had a higher number of sex partners over their lifetime, were smokers, or reported ever having had sex with another woman. Other studies have identified additional risks for BV, including IUD use, hormonal contraception, smoking, menses, and chronic stress.

BV is found in up to 50% or more of women who are at high risk of HIV acquisition in sub-Saharan Africa, and is estimated to be associated with an almost two-fold increase in risk of HIV acquisition in women in several prospective studies.

SCIENCE REVISITED

Of 1,196 pregnant women followed prospectively in Malawi (sub-Saharan Africa), the risk of HIV seroconversion was directly proportional to increasingly abnormal vaginal bacteria as measured by Gram stain score. Critically, new data shows that BV in women infected with HIV confers an increased risk of HIV transmission to male sex partners. BV may elevate these risks in several ways, including upregulation of relevant T-cell populations by the high burden of associated vaginal anaerobes;

Sexually Transmitted Diseases, First Edition. Edited by Richard H. Beigi.

reduced levels of protective factors (defensins, secretory leukocyte protease inhibitor) and increased levels of inflammatory factors (certain cytokines); and loss of hydrogen peroxide, which is virucidal.

Clinical and microbiologic characteristics of BV

In women of reproductive age, a vaginal environment that is quantitatively dominated by hydrogen peroxide (H_2O_2)-producing *Lactobacillus* species typically has a pH that is considered normal (<4.7), and has consistently been associated with healthy pregnancy outcomes, lack of abnormal vaginal symptoms, and reduced risk for acquiring several sexually transmitted pathogens, including HIV. The most commonly isolated *Lactobacillus* species associated with this healthy environment are *L. crispatus* and *L. jensenii*. These lactobacilli are autoinhibited by high levels of H_2O_2, so that the levels of H_2O_2-generating lactobacilli are self-regulated in the vagina.

Symptomatic BV, which accounts for approximately 60% of all cases, typically causes an abnormal vaginal discharge that is increased in amount and often malodorous. The odor, usually described as "fishy," is derived from volatilization

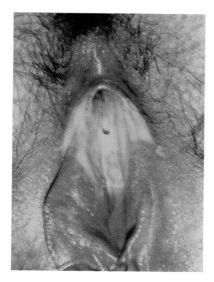

Figure 7.1. Typical vaginal discharge caused by bacterial vaginosis.

of the amines produced by the metabolism of anaerobic bacteria that characterize this disorder. The profound increase in anaerobe concentrations is characterized by the enhanced production of sialidase (which degrades IgA), glycosidase, volatile amines, and a characteristic cytokine profile. The elevation in sialidase forms the basis for one point-of-care rapid diagnostic test, BVBlue®.

Conventional cultivation of bacteria from vaginal fluid of women with BV typically yields a spectrum of primarily anaerobic commensals: *Gardnerella vaginalis*, *Prevotella* species, anaerobic Gram-positive cocci, *Mobiluncus* species, *Ureaplasma urealyticum*, and *Mycoplasma hominis*. More recently, molecular techniques that bypass cultivation requirements have been employed to greatly expand the microbiologic spectrum of BV. In addition to confirming the presence of previously described cultivatable BV-associated bacteria, these studies have detected *Atopobium vaginae*, *Lactobacillus iners*, *Eggerthella*, *Megasphaera*, *Leptotrichia*, *Dialister*, *Bifidobacterium*, *Slackia*, and bacteria related to *Arthrobacter*, *Caulobacter*, and *Butyrivibrio*. They have also detected several newly described bacteria in the *Clostridiales* order that are currently designated BVAB1, BVAB2, and BVAB3.

Critically, the initial event leading to the shift to the anaerobic predominance that characterizes BV is unknown, though data suggest that sex probably contributes — at least in some women. BV occurs more frequently among women who report new or higher numbers of male sex partners, is common and highly concordant among female sex partners, and rarely occurs before sexual debut – patterns that mimic the epidemiology of a typical sexually transmitted infection.

Evidence supports a role for male partners in the pathogenesis of BV, as some BV-associated bacteria, including *G. vaginalis*, *A. vaginae*, BVAB1, and *Megasphaera* type 1, have been detected in the partners of women with BV, with highest quantities in coronal sulcus swab samples; concentrations of these bacteria were low or undetectable in specimens from women without BV and from their male partners. The use of condoms to prevent BV is discussed below.

High BV prevalence (27% to 52%) in lesbians, and concordance of BV status in female couples, also support a role for sexual transmission. Sexual practices that transmit vaginal fluid between women increase the risk of BV. Gardner failed to causally implicate *G. vaginalis* after inoculating it into the vagina in 13 healthy women, as only one developed BV. However, 11 of 15 women developed BV when inoculated with the vaginal fluid of women with BV, suggesting transmissible factors. The practice of receptive oral sex has also been suggested as a risk for BV or "unstable" vaginal flora. These data support roles for exogenous (sexual acquisition) factors in the initiation and/or maintenance of BV.

Complications associated with BV

BV is associated with serious sequelae related to the upper genital tract, increasing the risk of preterm delivery, first trimester miscarriage in women undergoing in vitro fertilization, amniotic fluid infections, chorioamnionitis, postpartum and postabortal endometritis, and postabortal pelvic inflammatory disease (PID). In nonpregnant women, BV increases the risk of posthysterectomy infections and PID. BV itself may be associated with endocervical inflammation that manifests as mucopurulent cervicitis. Among HIV-infected women, the quantity of HIV shed in vaginal secretions from those with BV was increased nearly six-fold increase relative to those without BV. BV probably enhances women's likelihood of sexual acquisition of HIV, possibly through inducing reversible changes in the cervical or other mucosal immune environment. The exact means by which BV affects adverse reproductive tract sequelae is not clear. Possible explanations include loss of antimicrobial compounds produced by lactobacilli, destruction of mucin gel coating the vaginal/cervical epithelium via inhibition of glycosidase-producing anaerobes, degradation of local natural immune defenses, induction of a cervical pro-inflammatory environment, and alteration in the immune cell environment of the cervix.

Diagnosis

In clinical practice, BV is classically diagnosed using the Amsel criteria, which include the presence of at least three of four findings: a vaginal pH greater than 4.5; a homogeneous vaginal discharge on examination; detection of a fishy odor on the addition of potassium hydroxide to vaginal fluid (positive "whiff test"), and the presence of significant clue cells (defined as >20% of the total vaginal epithelial cells seen on 100× magnification on saline microscopy; see Figure 7.2). Other point-of-care diagnostic tests take advantage of immediate methods of detecting either high concentrations of *Gardnerella vaginalis* (the AFFIRM® test), a variety of the amines that are prominent, including sialidase (BVBlue®), trimethylamine, and prolineaminopeptidase, or some combination of amines, abnormal pH, and/or bacterial quantity (FemExam®). Despite the ease of use of these tests, clinicians often do not regularly pursue a specific diagnosis of vulvovaginal complaints, and rely (often inaccurately) on syndromic management to direct treatment. Moreover, the accuracy of the Amsel criteria in clinical practice is probably reduced by the limited skills in the use of microscopy to detect clue cells and rule out other important findings, including trichomonads and yeast forms. These skills can be improved by continued use of these tools by clinicians in the office setting.

BV may also be diagnosed using a score applied to Gram stains of vaginal fluid, the Nugent criteria, which quantifies the number of lactobacilli relative to BV-associated bacterial morphotypes to create a scale of flora abnormality ranging from normal (score = 0–3) through intermediate (score = 4–6) to frank BV (score = 7–10) (Figure 7.3). The Nugent score is widely regarded as the gold standard for the diagnosis of BV in research studies. Most recently, targeted qualitative and quantitative polymerase chain reaction (PCR) assays for the detection of various BV-associated bacteria have been studied, and although this approach may offer some utility in the future, it has not been widely validated for diagnosis of BV in large, diverse populations of women, and is costly. Moreover, quantitative PCR has not yet been well studied for its ability to differentiate between women who have intermediate flora vs. frank BV, as determined by the Nugent score. Women with intermediate flora by a Nugent score may have relatively high quantities of the BV-associated bacteria *G. vaginalis* and *A. vaginae* as determined by qPCR. The single commercially available panel using PCR

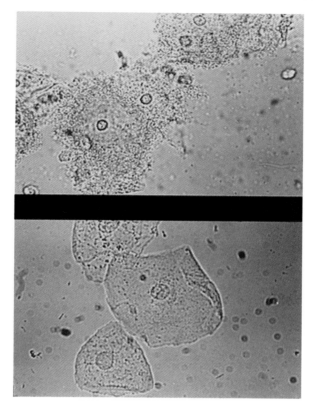

Figure 7.2. Saline microscopy of vaginal fluid showing numerous clue cells in a woman with bacterial vaginosis.

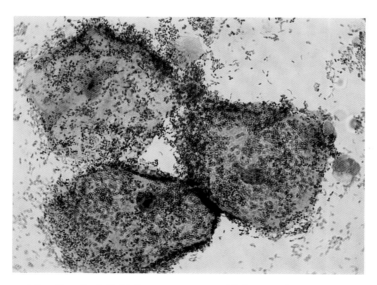

Figure 7.3. Gram stain of vaginal fluid from a woman with bacterial vaginosis. (Courtesy of Lorna Rabe, Magee-Womens Research Institute, Pittsburgh, PA, USA.)

offers detection of *G. vaginalis*, *Bacteroides fragilis*, *Mobiluncus mulieris*, and *M. curtisii*, and thus detects only a small proportion of the bacterial species that characterize BV. The optimal molecular methodology or criteria, both qualitatively and quantitatively, to serve as the next generation diagnostic modality has not been determined and thus is not currently recommended.

Cultures for *G. vaginalis* should not be used to diagnose BV because 36–55% of women without BV will harbor this organism as part of normal flora. *G. vaginalis* can be recovered at high concentrations – a million organisms or copies (using PCR assays) per milliliter of vaginal fluid – even in women lacking clinical signs or symptoms of bacterial vaginosis. Women with BV generally have 100 million organisms/mL of vaginal discharge.

Treatment and prevention of BV

Efforts to optimize the management of BV have been limited by a lack of knowledge about the etiology of the initial decline of hydrogen peroxide-producing lactobacilli that precedes the increase in vaginal anaerobes. Because the inciting event is not known, treatment of BV aims to reduce the vaginal burden of these anaerobes and to ameliorate concomitant symptoms of abnormal or malodorous vaginal discharge. Traditional pharmacologic treatment for episodic BV, detailed in Table 7.1, includes oral or intravaginal therapy with metronidazole or clindamycin. Both drugs are active against the majority of anaerobes that predominate in BV, and are relatively inactive at a clinically meaningful level against the desirable *Lactobacillus* species. The efficacy of oral and vaginal metronidazole is similar. With oral metronidazole given for 7 days, between 83% to 87% of women experience symptomatic improvement at 2 to 3 weeks. Improvement in vaginal symptoms occurs in 71% to 78% of women who use intravaginal metronidazole regimens; most available data refer to twice daily dosing, though a regimen of once daily dosing is used routinely and is recommended by the Centers for Disease Control and Prevention (CDC). A regimen consisting of metronidazole extended release tablets (750 mg) taken once daily for 7 days is also an FDA-approved regimen.

Table 7.1. Antibiotic treatment of non-pregnant women with BV

Recommended regimens

Metronidazole 500 mg orally[a] twice a day for 7 days

or

Metronidazole gel, 0.75%, one full applicator (5 g) intravaginally, once a day for 5 days

or

Clindamycin cream, 2%, one full applicator (5 g) intravaginally at bedtime for 7 days.[b]

Alternative regimens

Tinidazole 2 g orally[c] once daily for 2 days

or

Tinidazole 2 g orally once daily for 5 days

OR

Clindamycin 300 mg orally twice daily for 7 days

or

Clindamycin ovules 100 mg intravaginally once at bedtime for 3 days

[a] Patients should be advised to avoid consuming alcohol during treatment with oral metronidazole and for 24 hours thereafter.
[b] Clindamycin cream and ovules are oil-based and might weaken latex condoms and diaphragms (refer to clindamycin product labeling for additional information).
[c] Patients should be advised to avoid consuming alcohol during treatment with oral tinidazole and for 72 hours thereafter.

Efficacy of oral clindamycin has generally been equivalent to that of oral metronidazole, while vaginal clindamycin has sometimes produced somewhat lower cure rates than those of vaginal metronidazole regimens (48% in a recent multi-center study). However, not all studies have measured cure at similar times with the same criteria for cure.

Both clindamycin and metronidazole given orally are recommended for the treatment of BV throughout pregnancy (Table 7.2). Metronidazole vaginal gel can also be used, but most experts emphasize that systemic therapy is preferred. Cure rates in pregnancy are generally similar to those in nonpregnant women.

Table 7.2. Antibiotic treatment of pregnant women with BV

Metronidazole 500 mg orally twice a day for 7 days,
or
Metronidazole 250 mg orally three times a day for 7 days,
or
Clindamycin 300 mg orally twice a day for 7 days

Key issues

• BV represents a major imbalance in the ecology of the vagina, characterized by loss of hydrogen peroxide-producing *Lactobacillus* species (primarily *L. crispatus)* and concomitant overgrowth of commensal vaginal anaerobes, many of which cannot be grown using traditional culture methods and require molecular approaches.

• BV is the most common etiology of vaginal symptoms causing women to seek healthcare.

• Dysregulation of the mucosal immune system during BV is complex, and may facilitate the acquisition of other genital tract pathogens, including *Chlamydia trachomatis, Neisseria gonorrheae,* and HIV-1.

• Although antibiotics with potent activity against anaerobes often effect a short-term resolution of BV and its associated symptoms, rates of BV recurrence are very high.

• Cultures for *G. vaginalis* should not be used to diagnose BV because 36–55% of women without BV will harbor this organism as part of normal flora.

• Probiotics in the form of human vaginal lactobacilli are an inherently attractive means of treating BV, and are under study for this purpose.

Other antibiotics that have been used for the treatment of BV include triple sulfa cream given intravaginally for 7 days. In a recent study, improvement occurred in only 41% of women treated with this regimen; other data support this finding of low efficacy, thus triple sulfa cream is not recommended for treatment of BV.

Given the associated adverse outcomes, treatment of BV in pregnancy has received considerable attention. A meta-analysis of BV treatment trials in pregnant women included 10 studies that had enrolled 3,969 women. The authors concluded that treatment of BV effected a significant reduction in preterm delivery in high-risk patients who receive oral regimens with treatment durations of ≥ 7 days. For low-risk patients, the effects were nonsignificant. One recently published study demonstrated a significant reduction in preterm birth among 2,058 pregnant women offered treatment for BV relative to 2,097 not offered treatment (3.0% vs. 5.3%; $p = 0.001$). Whether all women should be tested for BV during pregnancy remains a matter of debate; most evidence weighs against it, and national guidelines recommend doing so only in the presence of symptoms of vaginitis.

Tinidazole, a nitroimidazole related to metronidazole, has been approved for the treatment of BV (as well as for trichomoniasis, giardiasis, and amebiasis). This drug is well absorbed, has a long half-life relative to that of metronidazole, and can be effective against metronidazole-resistant trichomoniasis. Cure rates for BV appear to be similar to those afforded by the metronidazole and clindamycin regimens.

SCIENCE REVISITED

The role of antibiotic resistance among BV-associated bacteria (BVAB) in promoting treatment failure is uncertain. Clindamycin-resistant bacteria have been reported among women treated with vaginal clindamycin, although this was not associated with reduced cure rates. Although *Mobiluncus* is often resistant to metronidazole, early studies indicated that women with *Mobiluncus* who were treated with metronidazole had the same rate of cure as women not colonized by *Mobiluncus*. In a recent prospective study, incidence of persistent BV at 30 days was 26%, and significantly higher in women with baseline detection of BVAB1, BVAB2, BVAB3, *Peptoniphilus lacrimalis* or *Megasphaera* phylotype 2. Detection of these bacteria at test-of-cure was associated with persistence, while post-treatment sexual activity was not. Taken together, these findings suggest that anaerobic Gram-negative rods have a more central role in the etiology of BV than *Gardnerella*, *Mobiluncus*, or the genital mycoplasmas.

Recurrent BV

While short-term response to standard treatment regimens is acceptable, symptomatic BV persists or recurs in 11–29% of women at 1 month and in 50–70% by 3 months. Long-term recurrence rates may approach 80% in certain populations. Possible reasons for this include: failure to continually suppress the growth of BV-associated bacteria; reinoculation with these organisms from an exogenous source (for example, sexually); persistence of host risk factors (for example, douching or use of an intrauterine device); failure to recolonize the vagina with H_2O_2-producing lactobacilli; and infection with a *Lactobacillus* phage that destroys vaginal lactobacilli. None of these mechanisms has been conclusively shown to explain the high rates of BV recurrence, or to identify women at increased risk for BV incidence, recurrence, or sequelae. However, evaluation of twice weekly suppressive vaginal metronidazole (0.75% gel used Monday and Thursday nights) is effective in suppressing BV, with the rationale being that suppression of vaginal anaerobic overgrowth may at least offer sustained relief from symptoms and eventually increase the chance of the vaginal physiology's return to normal.

Because BV recurrence is so common even with excellent anti-anaerobic antibiotic therapy, patients and investigators have attempted a wide range of other treatments. Commercially available *Lactobacillus* preparations do not contain lactobacilli that adhere to human vaginal epithelial cells, nor do they usually produce hydrogen peroxide, a probable key component for the protective benefit conferred by human vaginal lactobacilli. They are also frequently contaminated with other enteric organisms, presumably of bovine origin. For these reasons, neither oral nor intravaginal therapy with over-the-counter *Lactobacillus* preparations is recommended. Yogurt may contain several species of lactobacilli, but none adheres to vaginal epithelial cells or reliably produces hydrogen peroxide; thus, it has no role in BV treatment. Most recently, advances in the field of probiotics have infused new energy into therapeutic studies for BV. Probiotics are defined as "a product containing viable, defined microorganisms in sufficient numbers, which alter the microflora (by implantation or colonization) in a compartment of the host and by that exert beneficial health effects in this host." BV is a logical target for treatment with probiotics aimed at establishing sustained vaginal recolonization with appropriate *Lactobacillus* species. At least one human-derived strain of *Lactobacillus crispatus* is currently under study as a treatment for BV, but is not commercially available at this time.

Substances that act as vaginal acidifiers have been evaluated in small studies. BufferGel, a spermicidal microbicide that acidifies semen and vaginal fluid, showed a modestly beneficial effect, and is undergoing further study. However, another acidifier, Acijel, failed to effect an improvement in BV cure in one study, so the effects of these products may be unpredictable. Further, none offers a method to sustain low vaginal pH over time. However, an absorptive tampon that also releases lactic and citric acids has been approved by the FDA. Because this product was not categorized as a new drug, evidence to support any efficacy in preventing or treating BV was not included in the approval process. Finally, some investigators have recommended vaginal instillation of H_2O_2, either as a douche or in a saturated tampon. Concerns with this approach include that it involves douching, a procedure that most experts feel should be generally discouraged, that simple application of H_2O_2 may produce short-term disinfection but will not sustain resolution of abnormal flora over time, and that H_2O_2-producing lactobacilli may be killed by high concentrations of H_2O_2. Nonoxynol-9, a surfactant that can act as a microbicide, has not been shown to be effective in preventing acquisition of, or in treating, BV or any other STI, including HIV, and is not recommended.

Prevention of BV

Incorporation of our knowledge about key risk factors into client-centered counseling is likely to positively impact women's ability to prevent future episodes. First, douching is a major risk factor for BV, and for the loss of the vaginal lactobacilli that are associated with the clinical development of symptomatic BV. For this reason, because douching has also been epidemiologically linked to PID, ectopic pregnancy, and chlamydial cervical infection, and because douching provides no known prophylactic benefit against genital tract infection, women should be advised not to douche. The observation that BV is associated with the acquisition of a new sex partner, multiple sex partners, and sex with a female partner, implies that the use of barrier methods (condoms) may protect against its acquisition and against its persistence or recurrence if they are used in the first month after treatment for BV. Also, women who share vaginal sex toys should either use condoms on these toys between shared use, or wash thoroughly. Finally, limited data suggests a role for receptive anal and oral sexual behaviors; limiting these behaviors around the time of BV treatment might offer some protection, though data in this area is lacking.

⚠ SCIENCE REVISITED

Wives of men who participated in a randomized trial of circumcision to prevent HIV acquisition in Uganda were followed to assess the effects on vaginal infections. Among women without BV at enrollment, BV at follow-up was significantly less common in wives of men who had been circumcised compared to wives of men who had not (prevalence risk ratio (PRR) 0.80; 95% CI: 0.65–0.97). In women with BV at enrollment, persistent BV at one year was significantly lower in the circumcision-arm than the control-arm women (PRR 0.83; 95% CI: 0.72–0.96). Assessment of local bacteria pre- and post-circumcision among 12 participants revealed not only that several anaerobic bacterial families were detected in the subprepuceal space, but that they were significantly decreased in quantity and species diversity after circumcision.

Despite this intriguing data, several placebo-controlled trials have demonstrated that treatment of the male partner(s) does not improve the clinical outcome of the treatment of BV, or reduce its recurrence. The discrepancy between data suggesting the sexual acquisition of BV, and the lack of benefit of treating the male partner, remains puzzling, but does not rule out a role for sexual transmission. Part of the issue may be that the selection or dosing of the antibiotics used in the trials done to date was not appropriate or adequate for eradicating a potential reservoir for BV-associated bacteria in men.

The routine follow-up of women after treatment for BV is not recommended unless symptoms reappear.

Conclusion

Despite considerable research effort and recent advances, BV remains an enigmatic condition. Efforts to link BV to a single cultivated bacterial pathogen, such as *Gardnerella vaginalis*, have been unconvincing. Molecular tools have achieved some inroads. For one, they have revealed the complex microbiology of BV, expanding the spectrum even farther than was possible with cultivation-based approaches. However, it is possible that even with the more advanced technology, we are still missing key species. Some of the newly defined BV-associated bacteria do have very high specificity for BV, suggesting that they may play some critical role, but they do not appear to function as credible single causal pathogens. Numerous key questions still remain. What are the critical steps in the causal pathway to developing BV? What accounts for the high recurrence rate? Are all BVABs susceptible to antibiotics used to treat BV? Is biofilm formation critical to pathogenesis in BV? Finally, and critically: Are some communities or species of BVAB more pathogenic – for example, more strongly associated with adverse sequelae, such as preterm delivery – than others?

BV is most likely a heterogeneous syndrome caused by different communities of vaginal bacteria, similar to what occurs in conditions such as periodontitis linked to changes in oral microbial communities. In this sense, BV probably represents a dysbiotic condition caused not by a single pathogen but by a change in microbial composition and community structure. A woman's individual risk for acquiring a particular etiologic vaginal bacterial community might depend on specific practices, such as unprotected vaginal or oral sex. Future studies of BV will need to emphasize frequent prospective sampling for the vaginal microbiota, with careful attention to concurrent sexual and hygienic practices and, ultimately, innate characteristics of host immunity. The characterization of extravaginal reservoirs for BVAB – including the rectum and oropharynx – should also shed considerable light on the routes by which these bacteria establish dominance in BV.

★ TIPS & TRICKS

Examination for vaginitis
The evaluation of patients with suspected vaginitis rests mainly upon a physical examination of the vulva, vagina, and the discharge, and upon a microscopic examination of the discharge and determination of its pH. The amount, consistency, and location of the discharge within the vagina should be noted. In the absence of examination, some point-of-care tests can detect the most common pathogens associated with vaginitis, but the opportunity to assess the cervix as a source of discharge is lost; this may be critical in women at risk for cervical infection with gonorrhea or chlamydia.

1. Examine the external and internal labia for any signs, including fissures, edema, or erythema (all consistent with vulvovaginal candidiasis, genital herpes, or alternative noninfectious diagnosis).
2. Remove a sample of the discharge from the lateral vaginal wall with a swab, avoiding contamination with cervical mucus.

- Note its color in comparison with the white background of the swab.
- Determine pH directly by rolling the swab onto pH indicator paper. The pH of normal vaginal fluid is in the range of 4.0–4.5.

3. Take an additional specimen with another swab and mix separately into a drop of saline and a drop of 10% KOH on a microscope slide. Place a separate coverslip on the saline and KOH wet preps for microscopic examination.

Bibliography

Amsel R, Totten PA, Spiegel CA, et al. Nonspecific vaginitis. Diagnostic criteria and microbial and epidemiologic associations. *Am J Med* 1983; **74**: 14–22.

Brotman RM, Klebanoff MA, Nansel TR, et al. A longitudinal study of vaginal douching and bacterial vaginosis – a marginal structural modeling analysis. *Am J Epidemiol* 2008; **168**: 188–196.

Centers for Disease Control and Prevention. Sexually transmitted disease treatment guidelines, 2010. *MMWR* 2010; RR-12.

Koumans EH, Sternberg M, Bruce C, et al. The prevalence of bacterial vaginosis in the United States, 2001–2004; associations with symptoms, sexual behaviors, and reproductive health. *Sex Transm Dis* 2007; **34**: 864–869.

Fredricks DN, Fiedler TL, Marrazzo JM. Molecular identification of bacteria associated with bacterial vaginosis. *New Engl J Med* 2005; **353**: 1899–1911.

Fredricks DN, Fiedler TL, Thomas KK, et al. Targeted PCR for detection of vaginal bacteria associated with bacterial vaginosis. *J Clin Microbiol* 2007; **45**: 3270–3276.

Gray RH, Kigozi G, Serwadda D, et al. The effects of male circumcision on female partners' genital tract symptoms and vaginal infections in a randomized trial in Rakai, Uganda. *Am J Obstet Gynecol* 2009; **200**: 42 e1–7.

Hillier SL, Marrazzo JM, Holmes KK. Bacterial vaginosis. In: *Sexually Transmitted Diseases,*

4th edn. (Holmes KK,et al., eds.). McGraw-Hill; New York, 2008; pp. 737–768.

Marrazzo JM, Martin DH, Watts DH, et al. Bacterial vaginosis: identifying research gaps. Proceedings of a Workshop Sponsored by DHHS/NIH/NIAID. *Sex Transm Dis* 2010; **37**: 732–744.

Nugent RP, Krohn MA, Hillier SL. Reliability of diagnosing bacterial vaginosis is improved by a standardized method of gram stain interpretation. *J Clin Microbiol* 1991; **29**: 297–301.

Sobel J. Current concepts: vaginitis. *New Engl J Med* 1997; **337**: 1896–1903.

Sobel JD, Ferris D, Schwebke J, et al. Suppressive antibacterial therapy with 0.75% metronidazole vaginal gel to prevent recurrent bacterial vaginosis. *Am J Obstet Gynecol* 2006; **194**: 1283–1289.

US Preventive Services Task Force. Screening for bacterial vaginosis in pregnancy to prevent preterm delivery: USPSTF recommendation. *Ann Intern Med* 2008; **148**: 214–219.

Wiesenfeld HC, Hillier SL, Krohn MA, et al. Bacterial vaginosis is a strong predictor of *Neisseria gonorrhoeae* and *Chlamydia trachomatis* infection. *Clin Infect Dis* 2003; **36**: 663–668.

8

Trichomonas Vaginalis

Ravindu Gunatilake and R. Phillips Heine

Maternal-Fetal Medicine, Duke University School of Medicine, Durham, NC, USA

Introduction

Trichomonas vaginalis (TV) is the most common nonviral sexually transmitted infection (STI) world wide. Although a great majority of women can remain asymptomatic, TV infection can result in significant clinical consequences. Several complications associated with the reproductive period such as tubal infertility, premature rupture of membranes, low birth weight, and preterm delivery are all seen with greater frequency in the presence of TV. While the clinical diagnosis of TV remains imprecise, newer point-of-care testing based on molecular amplification methods combined with a keen recognition for treatment failure and appropriate management steps can help to mitigate these adverse effects. This chapter is specifically designed to provide the clinician with practical information on the basic pathology, diagnostic challenges, and therapeutic advances to optimally manage the patient infected with TV.

Epidemiology and risk factors

Trichomonas vaginalis was first discovered by Alfred Donne in 1836. Armed with the novel technology of microscopic examination, he noticed the presence of motile microorganisms in women with frothy vaginal discharge and pruritus. Centuries later, TV infection remains a prominent public health burden. The US Centers for Disease Control (CDC) estimates that TV infects

approximately 5 million individuals in the United States every year. The lack of current reporting requirements by US and international public health organizations underlies the challenge of estimating the true worldwide prevalence of TV. Despite this predictive challenge, the World Health Organization (WHO) estimates that there are over 170 million cases of trichomoniasis worldwide. This prevalence of TV is highly variable by geographic location and significant disparity exists in the rate of diagnosis and treatment of TV between developing and developed countries, favoring a higher disease burden in resource poor settings. Unlike other STIs in which the greatest prevalence exists in younger reproductive age women (ages 16–25), comparative studies of accurate molecular amplification testing in "low risk" populations have revealed that the highest rate of TV infection is typically found in older women (ages 36–40). TV is equally prevalent during pregnancy; however, subclinical infection rates of up to 95% have been reported in some US prenatal populations. Whereas there are few widespread prevalence studies of TV in women, there are even fewer epidemiological studies described in males. In most instances, males are unaware of their infection status and may serve as an asymptomatic reservoir, readily retransmitting TV to a previously treated partner.

Any sexually active female may acquire TV. However, an infected partner, low socioeconomic

Sexually Transmitted Diseases, First Edition. Edited by Richard H. Beigi.
© 2012 John Wiley & Sons, Ltd. Published 2012 by John Wiley & Sons, Ltd.

background, substance abuse, a history of bacterial vaginosis, and high-risk sexual practices (unprotected sex, multiple partners) are all cited as risk factors. In particular, female sexual workers who do not use condoms are at especially high risk for reinfection and may serve as a community reservoir for TV. This potential reservoir stands as an obstacle to any broad-based community treatment program for TV and, rather, argues for the development of a widespread vaccination program. It is important to note that these risk factors are not unique to TV, but are commonly associated with other STIs.

Pathology

TV is a flagellated parasitic protozoan, which reproduces by binary fission. It is typically pyriform or sometimes ameboid in shape with a primarily anaerobic life cycle. Humans are the only natural host for *Trichomonas vaginalis*, which solely infects the mucosal surfaces of the vagina, urethra, and prostate. Additional species of trichomonas (*Trichomonas tenax* and *Pentatrichomonas hominis*) that infect humans do not cause any significant illness. Studies suggest that TV is a very hearty organism, withstanding the harsh acidic environment of the vagina. It voraciously phagocytoses vaginal epithelial cells, bacteria, and erythrocytes. Following TV infection, through the release of various cytotoxic molecules, TV causes damage and sloughing of vaginal epithelial cells, and rapidly eradicates the predominant *Lactobacillus* species. TV also engages in mimicry, coating itself with host proteins, in the hope of avoiding the host immune system. Human to human transmission of TV trophozoites occurs via sexual intercourse while nonsexual transmission is exceedingly rare. It is important to note that the symptomatic presentation of TV infection is not unique. An array of alternative microorganisms must be considered in a woman presenting with vaginal symptoms. *Chlamydia trachomatis*, *Neisseria gonorrhea*, *Candida albicans,* and the altered flora of bacterial vaginosis "BV," with relative overgrowth of *Gardernella vaginalis*, *Mycoplasma hominis*, and anaerobic Gram-negative rods should be considered in the differential diagnosis.

Trichomonas and HIV

Similar to other STIs, such as gonorrhea and chlamydia, trichomoniasis also increases the propensity for HIV infection with studies suggesting a relative risk of 1.5–3 for acquiring HIV in the presence of TV coinfection. Considering the complexity of interactions between TV and vaginal epithelium, several molecular mechanisms have been proposed to account for this association between TV and HIV infection. TV can result in increased vaginal pH by eradicating normal vaginal flora as well as disrupting vaginal epithelium, thereby leading to the formation of small mucosal hemorrhages. The resulting change in the vaginal microbiome and epithelial damage may increase accessibility of HIV to the underlying vaginal tissue. TV infection also leads to a local inflammatory response, which may in fact predispose to HIV acquisition by the recruitment of CD4+ T cells, which are most susceptible to HIV infection. Studies have also suggested that the presence of TV delays the resolution of cervical HPV infection. The impact of this delay on the natural history of cervical dysplasia is unknown.

Trichomonas and pregnancy

The full spectrum of perinatal risk associated with TV infection during pregnancy is probably unknown. Nevertheless, a growing body of evidence has implicated TV with preterm delivery. Even after controlling for demographic and clinical variables, a large multicenter study found that TV was significantly associated with premature rupture of membranes (PROM), low birth weight, and preterm delivery. In another study, rates of PROM among patients with TV at term were approximately double the rates of PROM in patients without TV. The mechanisms for this association remain largely unknown, though the release of proinflammatory cytokines following TV infection has been proposed as a leading hypothesis. In a large inner city pregnant population, symptomatic TV was associated with higher concentrations of vaginal fluid white blood cells (WBCs). Further supporting this hypothesis, proinflammatory cytokines such as Interleukin 1,6, and TNF-alpha within both amniotic fluid and vaginal secretions have been found in higher concentration among women

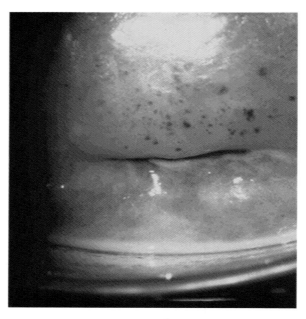

Figure 8.1. Strawberry cervix.

who ultimately delivered prematurely. While these previous studies support the biological plausibility of TV infection and premature delivery, further studies are needed to clarify the specific link.

Clinical presentation

Women with TV infection report a wide constellation of symptoms and there is no single pathognomonic presentation. When clinically apparent, symptoms often include vaginal pruritus, dysuria, dyspareunia, and a malodorous discharge. More severe infections may occasionally be associated with vulvitis and vaginitis. The characterization of vaginal discharge in the presence of TV infection is typically green-yellow and "frothy." Colpitis macularis or "strawberry cervix," reflecting cervical inflammation, may also be present on physical examination in approximately 5% of women with TV (Figure 8.1). However, it is important to keep in mind that approximately *50% of women with TV will be asymptomatic* at any given time. Table 8.1 illustrates the wide range of clinical symptomatology associated with TV infection. Unlike women, the spectrum of clinical infection in males is poorly characterized, though it is thought that greater than 75% of men are asymptomatic. Infre-

quently, trichomoniasis has been shown to cause urethritis, cystitis, epididymo-orchitis, and prostatitis in symptomatic males. In further contrast to females in whom TV infection festers for chronic periods of time, trichomoniasis in men often resolves relatively rapidly without treatment, typically resolving in approximately 2 to 16 weeks. TV reinfection occurs with significant frequency, which underscores the importance of consider-

Table 8.1. *Trichomonas vaginalis:* Signs and symptoms in females

Vaginal discharge – green to brown color (40%)

Malodorous discharge (50%)

Erythema or edema (20–40%)

Vaginal pruritus

Colpitis macularis "strawberry cervix" (5%)

Dysuria

Abdominal pain

Elevated vaginal pH > 4.5

Vaginal WBCs, amines, purulent discharge, vulvar erythema

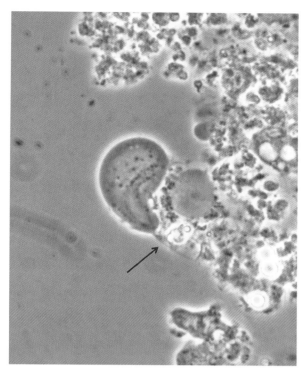

Figure 8.2. Vaginal wet mount (x 800) showing a trichomonas in the center with flagellae anteriorly (arrow). There is cellular debris and polymorphs in the right top corner. (Reproduced from Rogstad, K.E. et al. *ABC of Sexually Transmitted Infections*, 6th edn. Blackwell Publishing: Oxford, 2011, with permission.)

ation for rescreening at 3–6 months post-treatment or in the presence of recurrent symptomatology.

Diagnosis

There are no pathognomonic clinical signs or symptoms of *Trichomonas vaginalis* that preclude diagnostic testing. Current laboratory methods employed to diagnose TV include wet mount microscopy, culture, antigen detection, and a newly available nucleic acid amplification test (NAAT). Of these options, wet mount remains the most clinically utilized diagnostic technique, although the literature suggests it is an inferior test (Figure 8.2). When compared to the historical gold standard of vaginal swab cultures, sensitivities range from 60 to 80%. Sensitivities of microscopy are higher when the test is performed in symptomatic patients as well as in cases when the specimen is processed

immediately for viewing. A delay in processing of even 15 minutes will reduce the sensitivity. There is also a growing concern that decreased utilization of traditional microscopy has led to a failure in adequate training which will further decrease wet mount sensitivity outside of the research setting. The advantage of wet mount is that diagnosis can be accomplished at the point of contact, which allows for immediate therapy. Further, only one culture-based test is commercial available, in-pouch-TV™ (Biomed Diagnostics), which requires access to a laboratory with expertise in cultivation and microscopy.

Two point-of-care rapid antigen detection tests are currently available. OSOM TV™ (Genzyme Diagnostics) is a CLIA-waved point-of-care test indicated solely for the diagnosis of TV while the Affirm-VPIII (Becton–Dickinson) is a non-CLIA waived test that also tests for bacterial vaginosis and yeast infections. The OSOM TV™ test is more rapid (15 vs. 45 minutes) but requires separate tests to be performed for bacterial vaginosis (BV) and yeast. Sensitivities of both tests are superior to wet mount and equivalent to culture. Using an expanded gold standard incorporating NAAT, sensitivities of approximately 80–85% can be achieved for both tests. The advantages of these tests are the ease of processing and interpretation as well as the rapid availability of results. Prompt access to diagnostic results leads to point-of-care treatment, which greatly improves compliance and may offset the slight increase in sensitivity seen with NAAT.

The development of NAAT has enhanced the diagnosis of all sexually transmitted diseases including TV. In 2011, the APTIMA™ *Trichomonas vaginalis* assay (Genzyme) became the first nucleic acid test cleared by the Food and Drug Administration to diagnose TV. In studies comparing all four currently available techniques, sensitivities of NAAT approached 100%, while sensitivities of wet mount were approximately 50%. Increased sensitivity as well as ease of specimen handling and assay performance are the two major advantages of NAAT. Cost and delay in diagnosis, with subsequent delay in treatment, are the main impediments to widespread use.

⚠ CAUTION!

Wet mount is a suboptimal diagnostic test for trichomonas as it detects approximately 50% of infections. Additionally, a delay in processing a vaginal sample can lead to reduced sensitivity of testing.

Although not used as a primary diagnostic tool for the diagnosis of TV, the Pap smear has been utilized as a secondary screening test. The sensitivity of the Pap smear correlates well with wet mount microscopy, with liquid-based cytology testing being slightly superior to the standard Pap specimen processing. Conflicting data exists regarding the specificity of Pap testing, but most experts agree that confirmatory testing is appropriate, especially in low-prevalence populations.

A vaginal sample is the specimen of choice for all testing methodologies. As for all STD tests, the quality of the sample collected directly correlates with the sensitivity of the test. Urine sampling has been utilized for NAAT, but sensitivities are decreased compared to vaginal samples, making urine a suboptimal specimen in women being evaluated for TV. The advent of vaginal sampling has made patient self-collection a potential option for screening. Studies involving both point-of-care antigen detection testing as well as NAAT have demonstrated equivalent results when comparing patient-collected samples to those obtained by clinicians. As NAAT is based only on the presence of the organism and not on viability, screening programs utilizing patient collection with mail-in to a testing center may be ultimately possible. This patient-collected approach has been an effective screening strategy for *Neisseria gonorrhea* and *Chlamydia trachomatis* and will likely be appropriate for TV.

Management

Nitroimidazoles remain the only effective therapy for *Trichomonas vaginalis*. In the United States metronidazole and tinidazole are the two commercially available drugs. For the initial therapy of trichomonas, current CDC guidelines recommend a single 2 g oral dose of either drug. Both regimens have approximately 85–95% efficacy in treating initial trichomonal infections. If the patient has coexistent bacterial vaginosis, or has trouble tolerating the substantial one-time oral dose of therapy, extended therapy with 500 mg metronidazole administered orally twice a day for 7 days is recommended. This dose of metronidazole is also superior for the treatment of bacterial vaginosis than the single 2 g dose. Although not studied, it is likely that extended therapy with tinidazole would be equally effective for TV. In patients who do not respond to single-dose therapy, it is recommended that they either receive the extended 7-day therapy with metronidazole, or a single 2 g oral dose of tinidazole if metronidazole was the initial treatment drug. The provider should be aware that low levels of metronidazole resistance occur in approximately 2–5% of trichomonas isolates. Fortunately, most infections appear to respond to prolonged metronidazole therapy, or a single dose of tinidazole therapy. Tinidazole reaches higher vaginal concentrations than metronidazole, which may account for the improved efficacy among resistant infections.

In patients who fail to respond to this second course of therapy, an extended course of high-dose tinidazole or metronidazole at 2 g orally given twice a day for 5 days is recommended. Figure 8.3 details an algorithm to address treatment failure. Extended therapy is effective in approximately 80% of refractory patients. In the 20% of patients who fail therapy, expert consultation should be obtained. The Centers for Disease Control (CDC) website provides contact information and can arrange for sensitivity testing of the trichomonas isolate if deemed appropriate. Patients should be advised to avoid concomitant use of alcohol with nitroimidazoles as severe disulfiram-like reactions have been reported. Patients allergic to nitroimidazoles are rare, and if a true allergy is present, desensitization should be considered, as nitroimidazoles are the only effective therapy. Local therapy with metronidazole gel is not an appropriate therapy for TV. Cure rates with this treatment are less than 50%. This is likely secondary to infection of periurethral glands making vaginal therapy ineffective. Other topical agents, including mebendazole, paramomycin, or nonxynol-9 creams have been used with limited success. Their use should be limited to adjunctive therapy for refractory cases managed by a local infectious diseases expert.

★ TIPS & TRICKS

Single dose nitroimidazole therapy cures 85-95% of infections.

All patients infected with TV, and their sexual partners, should be treated. One particular population that deserves special consideration is the asymptomatic pregnant patient. Conflicting data exists regarding the impact of asymptomatic TV and pregnancy outcomes. In a randomized trial performed in the United States, the treatment of asymptomatic TV with two courses of metronidazole therapy increased the risk of preterm birth by approximately 50%. The majority of the increase in this study was limited to late preterm birth between 35 and 37 weeks gestation and there was concern regarding the adequacy of enrollment. A recent African study contradicts these findings in that therapy for *Trichomonas vaginalis* decreased the risk of preterm birth. Due to this conflicting data, as well as the pathology associated with *Trichomonas vaginalis* in the nonpregnant state, we recommend initiation of treatment at the time of diagnosis. If the decision is made to delay therapy, treatment should be initiated at approximately 35–37 weeks estimated gestational age as prematurity is no longer a concern. Partner treatment should not be delayed.

⚠ CAUTION

The use of nitromidazole can lead to a severe disulfiram-like reaction. Patients should be counseled to avoid alcohol during nitroimidazole therapy.

Metronidazole therapy is considered safe during any stage of pregnancy. In patients who are breastfeeding, it has been recommended that breastfeeding be discontinued for 24 to 72 hours after therapy in order to avoid neonatal exposure. This current recommendation appears potentially unfounded, however, as metronidazole is present in very low concentrations in neonatal blood, and safety during pregnancy has been well established.

Due to high efficacy of single-dose therapy, it is not recommended that patients with successful clinical treatment be given a test of cure. Rather, rescreening patients in 3–6 months should be considered, as approximately 20% of patients will become reinfected within this time period. As stated previously, patients infected with TV are at high risk for coinfection with other STIs or sexually-associated conditions, such as bacterial vaginosis. Diagnostic testing should also be performed for gonorrhea, chlamydia, syphilis, HIV, as well as bacterial vaginosis in conjunction with any diagnostic testing for TV. Vaccines for the prevention of hepatitis B and human papilloma

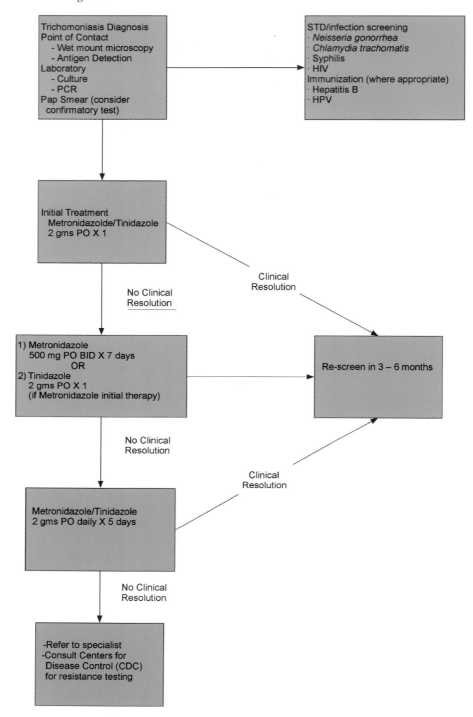

Figure 8.3. Trichomonas management flow chart.

virus (HPV) should also be recommended in the appropriate patient.

Conclusion

The epidemiological impact and clinical consequences of TV infection remain underappreciated. TV is a highly prevalent infection often lying dormant within an asymptomatic majority of affected women. Importantly, it is associated with perinatal complications and involved in the acquisition and transmission of HIV. With low-testing sensitivities, clinical symptoms and microscopy are inadequate for reliable diagnosis. Molecular amplification of *Trichomonas vaginalis* nucleic acids is now the modern gold standard for testing while rapid antigen detection is the most practical diagnostic test, enabling point-of-contact treatment. Single-dose nitroimidazole therapy cures the overwhelming majority (80–85%) of TV infection and the infrequent treatment failure can often be managed with prolonged oral therapy. Vaccine development appears to be a promising area of innovation and a future direction in management.

Bibliography

Andrea SB, Chapin KC. Comparison of Aptima Trichomonas vaginalis transcription-mediated amplification assay and BD affirm VPIII for detection of T. vaginalis in symptomatic women: performance parameters and epidemiological implications. *J Clin Microbiol* 2011; **49**(3): 866–869. PMCID: 3067695.

Cudmore SL, Delgaty KL, Hayward-McClelland SF, et al. Treatment of infections caused by metronidazole-resistant Trichomonas vaginalis. *Clin Microbiol Rev* 2004; **17**(4): 783–793, table of contents. PMCID: 523556.

Cudmore SL, Garber GE. Prevention or treatment: the benefits of Trichomonas vaginalis vaccine. *J Infect Public Health* 2010; **3**(2): 47–53.

Harp DF, Chowdhury I. Trichomoniasis: evaluation to execution. *Eur J Obstet Gynecol Reprod Biol* 2011; 157 (1): 3-9. Heine RP, McGregor JA, Patterson E, et al. *Trichomonas vaginalis*: diagnosis and clinical characteristics in pregnancy. *Infect Dis Obstet Gynecol* 1994; **1**(5): 228–234. PMCID: 2366141.

Heisterberg L, Branebjerg PE. Blood and milk concentrations of metronidazole in mothers and infants. *J Perinat Med* 1983; **11**(2): 114–120.

Huppert JS, Hesse E, Kim G, et al. Adolescent women can perform a point-of-care test for trichomoniasis as accurately as clinicians. *Sex Transm Infect* 2010; **86**(7): 514–519.

Huppert JS, Mortensen JE, Reed JL, et al. Rapid antigen testing compares favorably with transcription-mediated amplification assay for the detection of Trichomonas vaginalis in young women. *Clin Infect Dis* 2007; **45**(2): 194–198.

Lowe NK, Neal JL, Ryan-Wenger NA. Accuracy of the clinical diagnosis of vaginitis compared with a DNA probe laboratory standard. *Obstet Gynecol* 2009; **113**(1): 89–95. PMCID: 2745984.

Nanda N, Michel RG, Kurdgelashvili G, Wendel KA. Trichomoniasis and its treatment. *Expert Rev Anti Infect Ther* 2006; **4**(1): 125–135.

Nye MB, Schwebke JR, Body BA. Comparison of APTIMA Trichomonas vaginalis transcription-mediated amplification to wet mount microscopy, culture, and polymerase chain reaction for diagnosis of trichomoniasis in men and women. *Am J Obstet Gynecol* 2009; **200**(2): **188** e1–7.

Schwebke JR, Burgess D. Trichomoniasis. *Clin Microbiol Rev* 2004; **17**(4): 794–803, table of contents. PMCID: 523559.

Sobel JD, Nyirjesy P, Brown W. Tinidazole therapy for metronidazole-resistant vaginal trichomoniasis. *Clin Infect Dis* 2001; **33**(8): 1341–1346.

Stringer E, Read JS, Hoffman I, et al. Treatment of trichomoniasis in pregnancy in sub-Saharan Africa does not appear to be associated with low birth weight or preterm birth. *S Afr Med J* 2010; **100**(1): 58–64. PMCID: 3090676.

Workowski KA, Berman S. Sexually transmitted diseases treatment guidelines, 2010. *MMWR Recomm Rep* 2010; **59** (RR-12): 1–110.

Vulvovaginal Candidiasis, Desquamative Inflammatory Vaginitis, and Atrophic Vaginitis

Jack D. Sobel

Division of Infectious Diseases, Wayne State University School of Medicine, Detroit, MI, USA

Introduction

Vulvovaginal symptoms are extremely common, and are a major reason many women seek healthcare. Vaginal symptoms include an abnormal discharge which may be caused by either vaginal or cervical infection or may be due to numerous noninfectious causes. Other common symptoms include vulvovaginal pruritus, irritation, discomfort, burning, genital malodor, and variable discomfort or pain during or following intercourse. The subjects of bacterial vaginosis and trichomoniasis are dealt with in other chapters. The various vaginal syndromes and etiologies are listed in Table 9.1, and Table 9.2 depicts the vulvar syndromes and the associated known common etiologies.

Women may perceive a change in normal vaginal discharge reflecting a qualitative or quantitative alteration. Clinicians should not trivialize and dismiss this complaint. Instead they should thoroughly evaluate the woman's symptoms by clinical examination and routine laboratory tests such as pH, microscopy and occasionally culture. Some patients have other comorbid disorders such as atopy, common dermatoses, e.g. eczema or psoriasis, which may also need to be addressed. While bacterial vaginosis, vulvovaginal candidiasis, and trichomonas vaginitis are the most common infectious entities causing vulvovaginitis, it should be emphasized that vulvovaginal symptoms are more frequently the result of noninfectious etiology. Clinicians should cease to restrict consideration of differential diagnosis of vulvovaginal symptoms considering only cervical or vaginal infection as the cause of symptomatology. Clinicians are required to reach a specific diagnosis and avoid empiricism. Prescribing empirical measures, including the use of steroids when no diagnosis is available, should be avoided. Syndromic medicine is not an acceptable standard of care in industrialized countries.

Candida vulvovaginitis

Epidemiology

Vulvovaginal candidiasis (VVC) is extremely common in adolescents and adults. Fifty percent of female university students will have at least one physician-diagnosed episode by the age of 25 and as many as 75% of premenopausal women report having had at least one episode and 45% of women have two or more episodes. VVC is less common in post-menopausal women, unless they are taking estrogen therapy. It is estimated

Sexually Transmitted Diseases, First Edition. Edited by Richard H. Beigi.
© 2012 John Wiley & Sons, Ltd. Published 2012 by John Wiley & Sons, Ltd.

Table 9.1. Vaginal syndromes and their etiologies

Type	Etiology
Infectious	
Bacterial vaginosis	Mixed *Gardnerella vaginalis*, anaerobes (prevotella, porphyromonas, bacteroides, fusobacterium, peptostreptococcus, mobiluncus), and genital mycoplasmas
Candida vulvovaginitis	90% *Candida albicans*, 10% non-*albicans Candida* species, rarely other fungi
Trichomoniasis	*Trichomonas vaginalis*
Rare bacterial	Group A streptococcus
Noninfectious	
Atrophic vaginitis	Post-menopausal, post-partum, post-anti-estrogen therapy
Contact vaginitis	Contact dermatitis (hypersensitivity)
Chemical irritant	Soaps, detergents, topical antimycotics
Allergic vaginitis	Allergens
Desquamative inflammatory vaginitis (DIV)	Unknown (Bacterial? Immune mechanism?)
Erosive lichen planus	Immune mechanisms
Collagen vascular diseases (SLE)	Vasculitis
Pemphigus and pemphigoid syndromes	Immune mechanisms

Table 9.2. Vulvar symptoms

Infection	Etiology
Infectious	
Candida vulvovaginitis	> 90% *Candida albicans*
Rare bacterial	Group A streptococcus
Noninfectious	
Desquamative inflammatory vaginitis (DIV)	Unknown
Contact vulvovaginitis	Menstrual pads
Chemical irritant vulvitis	Soaps, detergents
Allergic vaginitis	Allergens
Dermatitis	
– Psoriasis	
– Eczema	
– Seborrhea	
Dermatosis	
– Erosive lichen planus	
– Lichen sclerosus	

that 6–8% of adult women suffer from recurrent *Candida* vaginitis (RVVC) which translates into millions of women world wide. Recurrent *Candida* vulvovaginitis, or RVVC, is defined as four or more episodes in a given year. Epidemiologic data is incomplete however, for several reasons: (1) the diagnosis of VVC is nonreportable and therefore prevalence estimates rely mainly upon self-reported histories of diagnosis by the physician; (2) infection is routinely diagnosed without the benefit of microscopy or culture and as many as one half of the women given this diagnosis may have other conditions; and (3) the widespread use of over-the-counter (OTC) antifungal drugs makes epidemiological studies difficult to perform in most countries. Self-diagnosis and therefore self-therapy is prevalent.

Pathogenesis

Candida organisms probably gain access to the vagina via migration across the perianal area from the rectum. However, once colonization occurs, long-term colonization frequently persists for months and years. Following *Candida* colonization, the organisms persist in the presence of the normal protective vaginal flora without causing symptoms until additional precipitating factors alter the delicate relationship between the *Candida* microorganisms and the vaginal microbiota as well as protective host defenses. A large number of underlying risk factors contribute to both colonization as well was symptomatic disease (Figure 9.1).

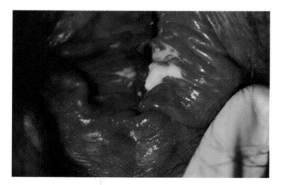

Figure 9.1. Typical clinical features of *Candida* vulvovaginitis with intense erythema and edema of the vestibule and vulva with an adherent "clumpy" white discharge.

Microbiology

Candida albicans is responsible for 90% or more of episodes of VVC. The remainder of the attacks are caused by non-*albicans Candida* species, which included *C. parapsilosis, C. glabrata, C. tropicalis,* and a variety of rare *Candida* species, an occasional non-*Candida* yeast *Saccharomyces* species. Some investigators have reported an increased frequency of the non-*albicans Candida* species, particularly *glabrata*, but this has not been confirmed. The non-*albicans Candida* species appear to be less virulent both in patients as well as in animal models used to study pathogenesis. Nevertheless, these species are still capable of causing symptomatic vaginitis, although their causal role needs to be established in each given patient. Accordingly, all *Candida* species produce similar vulvovaginal symptoms, although the severity of symptoms appears to be milder with *C. parapsilosis* and *C. glabrata* as compared to *C. albicans.*

Risk factors

Sporadic attacks of VVC frequently occur without identifiable precipitating factors. Nevertheless, a number of factors do predispose to symptomatic infection:

- One-quarter to one-third of women are prone to VVC during or after taking broad spectrum antibiotics. No antibiotics, either systemic or local, are immune from this complication. The mechanism whereby antibiotics induce *Candida* vaginitis has not been fully established. Previously, it was thought that antibiotics inhibit bacterial flora primarily in the gastrointestinal tract or possibly within the vagina allowing the overgrowth of potential pathogens such as *Candida.* However, confirmation of this hypothesis is not available. Administration of lactobacillus (oral or vaginal) probiotics during or after taking antibiotic therapy does not prevent post-antibiotic VVC.
- Increased estrogen levels. VVC is rare before puberty and tends to be less frequent in the post-menopausal women not taking any form of exogenous estrogen. Similarly, symptoms tend to flare in the pre-menstrual period on a cyclical basis. VVC appears to be more common in the setting of increased estrogen levels

such as with oral contraceptives, especially when estrogen dose is high, pregnancy, and pre-menopausal estrogen therapy especially with topical use of estrogen.

- Diabetes mellitus. Women with diabetes, especially those with poor glycemic control, are more prone to VVC. In particular, women with type 2 diabetes appear to be prone to *C. glabrata* infections. Nevertheless, most women with RVVC do not suffer from diabetes, including chemical or pre-diabetes. Routine glucose tolerance tests are not indicated in women with VVC, either sporadic or recurrent.
- Immunosuppression. *Candida* infections are more common in immunosuppressed patients, especially those taking corticosteroids or with HIV infection.
- Contraceptive devices. Vaginal sponges, diaphragms, and IUDs have been associated with VVC in some studies. Spermicides are not thought to increase VVC.
- Genetic susceptibility. Although a genetic factor was suspected for many years, evidence confirming this relationship was not available until recently. Earlier, suspicions were based on a family history, and blood group, including blood secretor status. It is likely that more than one genetic factor is complicit in the pathogenesis of VVC. Genetic factors may be important in colonization, as well as in determining the immune response to the presence of proliferating organisms within the vagina. Accordingly, VVC has been reported with decreased in vivo concentrations of mannose binding lectin (MBL) and increased concentrations of IL-4. Two specific gene polymorphisms variance in the MBL and IL-4 genes can account for this finding in some high-risk women but their relevance remains controversial. The prevalence of a variant MLB gene is higher in women with RVV than in controls without candidiasis. Recognition of *C. albicans* by the innate hose defense system is mediated by pattern-recognition from the toll-like receptor (TLR) and lectin like-receptor families. Mannans from the Candida cell wall are recognized by the mannose receptor, and TLR4 and TLR2 recognize phospholipomannan and collaborate with the β-glucan receptors dectin-1 in the stimulation of cytokine production. Dectin-1 amplifies TLR2- and TLR4-induced cytokine production by human cells, including TNF and in addition IL-17, IL-6 and IL-10. Human dectin-1 deficiency as a causative factor in mucocutaneous fungal infection is now established.

- Behavioral factors. Although VVC is not considered a sexually transmitted disease (because it occurs in celibate women and *Candida* is considered part of the normal vaginal flora), this does not mean that the sexual transmission of *Candida* microorganisms does not occur, or that VVC is not associated with sexual activity. Accordingly, one observes an increase in the frequency of VVC at the time that most women begin regular sexual activity. Male partners of infected women are more likely to have penile colonization than partners of uninfected women, and usually with the same strain as indicated by strain typing.
- There is no high quality evidence showing the link between VVC and hygienic habits or in using tight or synthetic clothing.
- HIV infection. VVC occurs with higher incidence and greater persistence, but not greater severity, among HIV-infected women. A significantly increased rate of symptomatic infection is confined only to HIV-infected women with very low CD4 counts and very high viral load – a population likely to manifest other AIDS manifestations. HIV testing of women, only for the indication of recurrent VVC is not justified given that recurrent *Candida* vaginitis is a common condition in women without HIV infection and the majority of cases occur in HIV-uninfected women. Only women with risk factors for acquisition of HIV should be counseled and offered screening. The microbiology of recurrent VVC in HIV-infected women is the same as in HIV-negative women.
- *Candida* colonization of the vagina in asymptomatic women may persist for prolonged periods of time until precipitating exogenous factors trigger a change in the balance between host and pathogen. Triggering is most often the result of changes in the host, in which naturally occurring anti-*Candida* vaginal defensive mechanisms diminish or fail. *Candida* proliferation follows with increase in numbers of organisms and expression of virulence factors including hyphal formation and elaboration of

proteases. The development of symptoms and signs of vulvovaginal inflammation, however, usually requires the involvement of the host adaptive immune response reacting to the proliferating organisms. It is this latter response which is critical for the development of symptomatic VVC and may be seen as an unnecessary byproduct of the host defense system reacting to the organisms.

Clinical features

Vulvar pruritus is the dominant feature of VVC. Women may also complain of dysuria, often described as external rather than internal, irritation, soreness, and dyspareunia. There is often little or no discharge, and when present the discharge is typically white and clumpy. Physical examination reveals erythema of the vulva and vaginal mucosa with vulvar edema (Figure 9.1). The discharge is typically described as clumpy and cottage-cheese like. However, it may also be thin and watery, indistinguishable from the discharge of other forms of vaginitis. Some patients, particularly those with *C. glabrata* infection, have little discharge with only erythema on vaginal examination. The vulva is invariably involved and fissures may be present. It is important to recognize that, in contrast to bacterial vaginosis, *Candida* infection involves both vulva and vagina.

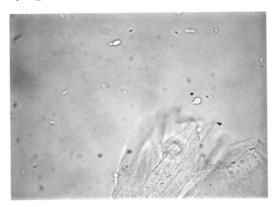

Figure 9.2. High-power wet mount microscopy revealing multiple budding yeast in the absence of polymorphonuclear or leukocytes or hyphal elements in a patient infected with *Candida glabrata*.

50% of patients with confirmed VVC. Empiric therapy is often considered with typical clinical findings, normal vaginal pH and no other pathogens visible on microscopy. However, with an unconfirmed microscopy-based diagnosis, a culture should be obtained. Often empiric therapy can be delayed until the results of additional tests are available. Cultures provide confirmation of the diagnosis within 48–72 hours and also reveal the species of the organism which facilitates the selection of the appropriate antifungal agent. Culture is most important and should be performed in all patients with persistent or recurrent symptoms, because many of these women have non-*albicans Candida* infections with reduced susceptibility to azoles. In the presence of positive microscopy and a normal pH, a routine culture is not essential, but should be done in microscopy-negative patients.

Low-risk commercial tests are now available as an alternative to culture. These include: (1) Affirm® test in which a DNA probe with hybridization is particularly useful and should provide results within several hours to confirm the initial clinical diagnosis. The Affirm® test also provides an opportunity to diagnose bacterial vaginosis or trichomoniasis. (2) PCR testing is widely available through commercial laboratories and is a highly sensitive method that provides *Candida* speciation when positive. The cost efficacy of the PCR

SCIENCE REVISITED

There appears to be a strong component of genetic susceptibility in terms of yeast colonization status as well as the immune response to that colonization.

Diagnosis

The vaginal pH is typically 4–4.5, which distinguishes VVC from trichomoniasis or bacterial vaginosis. The clinical diagnosis should be confirmed by finding the organism on saline wet mount microscopy and by adding 10% KOH, which facilitates the microscopic recognition of the yeast and hyphal morphotype (Figure 9.2). Unfortunately, microscopy may be negative in technology has not been evaluated and may take 48–72 hours for results, similar to microbial culture. Although PCR offers a more sensitive method of diagnosis, the clinical relevance of this increased sensitivity is unknown. Likewise, the significance of a positive PCR result after antimycotic therapy is unclear. A Pap smear is positive in approximately 25% of patients with culture-positive symptomatic VVC and is therefore of low sensitivity but of high positive predictive value.

The mere demonstration of the presence of *Candida* by any of the aforementioned diagnostic methods in no way confirms the pathogenic role of *Candida* in the specific patient or clinical syndrome. This is because *Candida* is found colonizing 15–20% of asymptomatic healthy women. Accordingly, the mere presence of *Candida* does not imply culpability. The determination of the causation of symptoms requires the exclusion of other pathogens, including the finding of a normal pH. No other infectious causes are responsible for vulvovaginal symptoms at normal pH 4.0–4.5.

> ★ TIPS & TRICKS
>
> Finding *Candida* without any associated symptoms does not warrant treatment, as roughly 15–20% of women are colonized by yeast at any one time.

Differential diagnosis

Other conditions should be considered in the differential diagnosis of symptomatic women with normal vaginal pH, and these include allergic and chemical reactions, hypersensitivity reactions, and contact dermatitis. These conditions are extremely common and frequently will cause symptoms in the presence or absence of *Candida*. If the vaginal pH exceeds 4.5 or excessive PMNs are present, mixed infections with bacterial vaginosis or trichomoniasis may be present. Based on the aforementioned criteria, there should be no difficulty separating bacterial vaginosis from *Candida* vaginitis. Self-diagnosis of VVC is frequently inaccurate. Similarly, diagnosis

of *Candida* vaginitis by telephone is unreliable and should not be performed.

> ★ TIPS & TRICKS
>
> Self-diagnosis and/or telephone diagnosis of vaginal yeast infections (and all vaginitis syndromes) is highly inaccurate and should not be done given the high possibility of mis-diagnosis and mismanagement.

Treatment

Treatment is indicated for the relief of vulvovaginal symptoms. There is no indication to treat asymptomatic colonization in culture-positive women. A number of highly effective oral and intravaginal antifungals are available (Table 9.1). Nystatin is the least effective with cure rates in the 70–75% range. The remaining antifungals have published efficacies in the 80–88% range. Of the intravaginal imidazoles, clotrimazole, miconazole, butoconazole, and tioconazoles are available over-the-counter (OTC) in the USA, while terconazole is available only by prescription. All these topical agents are highly effective and are prescribed as single-day to 7-day regimens. There appears to be no superiority of one regimen over another. Topical regimens are well tolerated with few adverse effects, although burning may occasionally occur. Mild disease is best treated with shorter dose regimens (Table 9.3).

Oral agents are available in the USA for the treatment of *Candida* vaginitis and include fluconazole which is supplied as a single 150 mg oral tablet, itraconazole and ketoconazole. Only fluconazole is FDA approved for VVC treatment.

Selection of the appropriate antifungal agent and the duration of therapy has been facilitated by the VVC classification complicated and uncomplicated VVC (Table 9.4). Most women (uncomplicated VVC) being healthy, hosts with mild to moderate, infrequent episodes of vaginitis due to *C. albicans*. In these circumstances, patients respond to all azoles, topical or systemic, with a success rate in excess of 90% regardless of duration of therapy.

Table 9.3. Therapy for vaginal candidiasis

Drug	Topical agents and formulation	Dosage regimen
Butoconazole[a]	2% cream	5 g × 3 d
Clotrimazolea[a]	1% cream	5 g × 7–14 d
	2% cream	5 g × 3 d
	100 mg vag tab	1 tab × 7 d
	100 mg vag tab	2 tab × 3 d
	500 mg vag tab	1 tab single dose
Miconazole[a]	2% cream	5 g × 7 d
	4% cream	5 g × 3 d
	100 mg vag supp.	1 supp. × 7 d
	200 mg vag supp.	1 supp. × 3 d
	1200 mg vag supp.	1 supp. single dose
Econazole	150 mg vag tab	1 tab × 3 d
Fenticonazole	2% cream	5 g × 7 d
Ticonazole[a]	2% cream	5 g × 7 d
	6.5% ointment	5 g single dose
Terconazole	0.4% cream	5 g × 7 d
	0.8% cream	5 g × 3 d
	80 mg vag supp.	80 mg × 3 d
Nystatin	100,000–U vag tab	1 tab × 14 d
	Oral agents	
Ketoconazole	400 mg bid	× 5 d
Itraconazole	200 mg bid	× 1 d
	200 mg	× 3 d
Fluconazole	150 mg	single dose

[a] OTC in the United States.
Abbreviations: vag, vaginal; tab, tablets; supp, suppository.

Table 9.4. Classification of vulvovaginal candidiasis

Uncomplicated	Complicated
Sporadic/infrequent VVC *and*	Recurrent VVC *or*
Mild to moderate VVC *and*	Severe VVC *or*
Likely to be *C. albicans* and	Non-*albicans* candidiasis *or*
Normal, nonpregnant host	Abnormal host, e.g. uncontrollable diabetes debilitation, immunosuppression

VVC = vulvovaginal candidiasis.

In contrast, women with complicated VVC respond less well to short course azole therapy. Accordingly, women with a compromised immune system and severe vaginitis should receive more prolonged, conventional antimycotic therapy, usually requiring up to 7 days of treatment. The treatment of women infected with non-*albicans Candida* species remains problematic. *C. krusei* infection is fortunately extremely rare and resistant to fluconazole, but responds rapidly to other azoles. Vaginitis due to *C. glabrata* is, however, refractory to all forms of azole therapy with only a 50% success rate. Somewhat improved results are achieved with vaginal boric acid, with 60–70% eradication rates. The best results follow vaginal therapy with 17% flucytosine cream. The latter has to be compounded, is not available commercially, and is extremely expensive in most settings. More important than selecting an antifungal agent is deciding whether to treat vulvovaginal symptoms in the presence of culture positive *C. glabrata*. The mere finding of *C. glabrata* does not imply complicity in the pathogenesis of the clinical syndrome. More often than not, *C. glabrata* is an innocent bystander and intensive treatment regimens directed at *C. glabrata* frequently fail. Moreover, even when successful, organism elimination is not accompanied by a concomitant relief or eradication of symptoms. In the experience of some investigators, less than 25% of the symptoms of symptomatic *C. glabrata* positive patients can be attributed to *C. glabrata* isolated. Nevertheless, when no other explanation for symptoms is available, a trial of therapy is clearly justified, but clinicians should not trivialize the complex relationship between this yeast and vulvovaginal symptoms.

Treatment of recurrent vulvovaginal candidiasis

As describe above, RVVC occurs in 5–8% of the female population during their reproductive period. It is likely that genetic factors are operative in the overwhelming majority of such patients. Nevertheless, secondary precipitating mechanisms are frequently present and vary from patient to patient. Thus, while all patients share an underlying genetic predisposition, triggers to symptomatic episodes vary considerably. Resistance of microorganisms to azole drugs is a rare cause of recurrent *Candida* vaginitis.

Before embarking on any treatment protocol, the diagnosis must be confirmed by the presence of culture, which includes organism speciation. Fungal susceptibility tests are not routinely indicated unless drug breakthrough infection or refractory disease occurs with appropriate azole therapy. Every effort should be made to control trigger mechanisms including the use of antibiotics, control of diabetes, and local predisposing factors such as concomitant vulvar dermatosis. Once these factors have been excluded or treated, an induction regimen with an antimycotic followed by a long-term suppressive maintenance regimen is indicated. While this can be accomplished with topical regimens, the duration and frequency of therapy suggests that oral therapy is more convenient and offers a more realistic solution. It should be emphasized that the therapy selected is aimed at controlling symptomatic episodes rather than guaranteeing that a cure will be achieved. The use of long-term suppressive maintenance regimens has been confirmed in several prospective controlled studies. Accordingly, after an induction regimen of fluconazole 150 mg given every 72 hours for 3 doses, a weekly maintenance regimen of fluconazole 150 mg once weekly is suggested. Complete resolution of symptoms follows within a matter of weeks, and the patient remains asymptomatic for the duration of therapy, which is recommended for 6 months. During this period, the patient invariably remains culture negative and asymptomatic. Following discontinuation of therapy after 6 months, approximately 50% of patients rapidly become recolonized and develop recurrent symptoms of VVC. However, 50% of patients will return to attack-free life with risks similar to low-risk women. Should symptomatic recurrence rapidly follow discontinuation of therapy, repeat re-induction and maintenance therapy is recommended this time for at least 12 months. Frequently, even longer prolonged maintenance regimens are recommended and required.

Atrophic vaginitis

Atrophic vaginitis, also called urogenital atrophy, refers to the extremely common condition that is characterized by atrophy of the vagina, vestibule, and vulva as a consequence of estrogen deficiency. The dominant target of estrogen deficiency is the vaginal epithelium which loses its rugosity and undergoes progressive thinning and atrophy. Simultaneously, but often less conspicuous, is progressive thinning of the vestibular epithelium. Atrophy of the vaginal epithelial lining is accompanied by reduced glycogen synthesis; this serves as a critical substrate for resident bacteria which break down glycogen to produce organic acid, most importantly lactic acid, further resulting in the loss of *Lactobacillus* species, the dominant component of vaginal microbiota. Accordingly, a consistent consequence of estrogen deficiency is the elevation of vaginal pH, usually above 5.0.

Low estrogen levels reduce vaginal secretions which result in vaginal dryness, but not infrequently, and paradoxically, a vaginal discharge is perceived to exist, or may in fact present as a watery discharge. Atrophic vaginitis typically occurs in menopausal women but it can also occur in women at any age who have a decrease in estrogenic stimulation to this area of the genitalia. In pre-menopausal women, hypoestrogenic settings include the post-partum, lactation, and during administration of anti-estrogenic drugs. Vaginal atrophy that follows the gradual decline in estrogen production is often associated with manifestations at other sites as well, including the bladder floor and urethra. Accordingly, urethral and bladder symptoms may be a manifestation of estrogen deficiency, including dysuria. Loss of estrogen also has an effect on the bladder lining, facilitating the development of bacterial cystitis in aging women. Another impact of estrogen deficiency relates to the loss of muscle tone, dilatation of the vaginal introitus, and contributes to the development of prolapse of bladder, uterus, and rectum.

Clinical manifestations

The earliest effects of estrogen deficiency are progressive atrophy and diminished vaginal secretions manifesting as vaginal dryness experienced during intercourse. While early symptoms may be relieved in part by the use of vaginal lubricants, invariably, progressive estrogen deficiency will not be compensated by the use of such lubricants. Ultimately, adequate vaginal lubrication for pain-free intercourse will require adequate estrogenic effect on the vaginal epithelium in many women. Vaginal dryness is often experienced by women long before the onset of amenorrhea or the development of systemic vasomotor symptoms and is often followed by dyspareunia. Dyspareunia is initially superficial or entry in nature, but with progression of the vaginal atrophy the discomfort will be experienced throughout, and following, intercourse, with discomfort and irritation and even itching lasting for several days after intercourse. With advanced atrophy, patients may complain of post-coital bleeding as a result of the susceptibility of the thinned vaginal epithelium to the effects of local friction and trauma.

Diagnosis

Vaginal atrophy and estrogen deficiency can be easily diagnosed without the use of sophisticated testing. The vaginal pH becomes elevated in excess of 4.5 and may reach levels in excess of 6. The vaginal pH is an excellent marker of estrogen deficiency. The elevated pH is a consequence of the loss of the lactic and other organic acid-producing bacteria. Lactic-acid-producing bacteria are replaced in part by Gram-negative organisms (usually coliforms) which in their own right are not pathogenic. On wet mount microscopy, the paucity of the typical rod-shaped bacterial morphotypes is apparent. Another important diagnostic feature is the appearance of parabasal epithelial cells reflecting a lack of maturation of basal and parabasal cells in the absence of adequate estrogen stimulation to achieve full maturation effect. It is unnecessary to request the maturation index that some labs offer. A simple increase in the number of parabasal cells will confirm the diagnosis of atrophic vaginitis in the presence of elevated pH and altered bacterial flora. It is also unnecessary and often misleading to measure serum estradiol levels. The latter test is redundant and does not parallel vaginal findings. It is important also to note that receipt of oral or transcutaneous estrogen products does not preclude the development of vaginal atrophy.

Treatment

One of the most remarkable biological phenomena is the reversible nature of vaginal atrophy. Following adequate estrogen replacement, especially by the vaginal route, a rapid transformation can be anticipated with reversal of the vaginal thinning together with reconstitution of healthy, protective bacterial flora with a dominant lactobacillus morphotype as well as the return to normal vaginal pH and accompanied by the disappearance of parabasal cells. This dramatic change can be expected within 4 to 6 weeks of adequate estrogen replacement therapy. A number of local vaginal treatments may be used to rectify atrophic vaginitis. These include intravaginal estradiol (Premarin®, Estrace®) as creams or vaginal suppositories of estradiol (Vagifem®). Alternatively intravaginal estriol may be used. While many practitioners rely on systemic estradiol to ensure vaginal health and prevent atrophy, not infrequently vaginal atrophy continues and progresses in the presence of systemic estrogen therapy. Accordingly, one should always use local intravaginal therapy for this diagnosis. A more recent alternative is the use of the estrogen-releasing vaginal rings of which several varieties are available. One can anticipate a return to vaginal health within 1 to 2 months, although the use of lubricants during intercourse may still be required and does not appear to have any negative implications.

★ TIPS & TRICKS

Treatment with vaginal estrogen is highly effective at ameliorating the symptoms of atrophic vaginitis, and should be undertaken in women with the characteristic clinical findings.

Desquamative inflammatory vaginitis (DIV)

Desquamative inflammatory vaginitis (DIV) is a relatively uncommon, chronic, clinical syndrome of unknown etiology, characterized by purulent vaginitis with variable findings in the vaginal, vestibular, and vulvar tissues.

Epidemiology

DIV occurs more frequently in peri-menopausal and post-menopausal women. Occasionally women may be seen in the fourth decade of life. This syndrome has been documented almost exclusively in Caucasian women. It is an extremely rare finding in African-American women and occurrence in Asian women is unknown. The unique findings in older women suggests a possible link to estrogen deficiency.

Pathogenesis

The cause of the syndrome remains unknown. Given the purulent nature of the vaginal discharge together with the increase of inflammatory cells, DIV was initially thought to be of infectious etiology. Numerous early studies using antibiotics, however, failed to show any benefit, suggesting an alternative causation. Subsequent-

ly, a dramatic response was shown to topical intravaginal 2% clindamycin, and the infectious causation theory was reborn. However, numerous attempts to identify a unique pathogen have not yielded any microbial clues or pathogens. Moreover, the excellent response that follows the use of topical steroids has once more forced investigators to consider a noninfectious etiology. Comorbidities such as autoimmune disorders have not been reported.

Clinical features

Women with DIV present with complaints of vaginal irritation, soreness, and dyspareunia lasting months and frequently years. The dominant complaint is that of a fairly profuse vaginal discharge which is described as brownish or yellowish-green in color. No malodor is associated with this discharge. Almost invariably, dyspareunia is present, which previously had been attributed by practitioners to estrogen deficiency or to unknown causes.

Patients are found to have a copious, purulent, yellowish discharge indistinguishable from that of trichomoniasis, except for the absence of malodor. Clinical findings, while almost invariably present in the vagina, frequently extend to the vestibule and vulva. A clinical spectrum exists which varies from diffuse erythema to focal, localized erythematous areas which are best seen as an annular erythematous rash. The rash is often most severe in the upper third of the vagina and on the neck of the cervix, resulting in an appearance similar to a "ure cervix"(Figure 9.3).

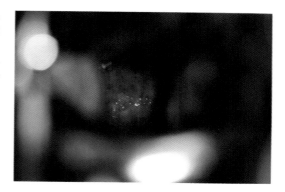

Figure 9.3. Erythematous annular vaginal lesions resembling a "strawberry" appearance in a patient with desquamative inflammatory vaginitis (DIV).

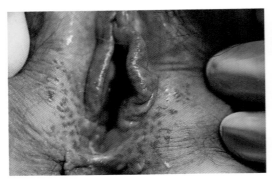

Figure 9.4. "Strawberry-like" rash of DIV involving labia minora and vulva.

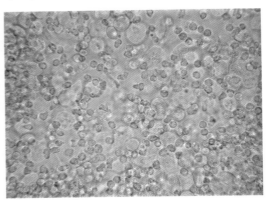

Figure 9.5. High-power saline microscopy revealing presence of inflammatory cells, both polymorphonuclear and mononuclear, and parabasal cells indicative of DIV.

This rash has been called both colpitis macularis or papular colpitis.

Although initially thought to represent focal, erosive or ulcerative changes, these annular lesions are now thought to represent a focal site of intense local inflammation resulting in the papular appearance. In addition to the annular lesions, occasional ecchymotic lesions are evident and particularly apparent in the vestibule. Other vaginal manifestations include erythematous linear changes resembling erythematous ridges. Nonspecific inflammatory changes involving the vestibule and the labia minora are frequently described in at least one-third of patients, and occasionally rash-like inflammatory changes are evident on the labia majora (Figure 9.4).

Diagnosis

The cardinal feature of DIV is the elevated vaginal pH in excess of 5 and frequently higher. On saline microscopy, there is an increase of inflammatory cells which vary from polymorphonuclear leukocytes (PMNs) to mononuclear cells. Invariably present is an increase of parabasal cells (Figure 9.5). Vaginal microbiota undergo major disruption which is evident as a mixed flora but clearly abnormal flora on wet mount microscopy. No additional diagnostic tests are currently available. The diagnosis is therefore clinical, based on the appearance of the purulent discharge, physical findings together with elevated pH, and inflammatory findings including the essential presence of parabasal cells. All the aforementioned criteria are required for a confident diagnosis.

Treatment

A study in 1993 reported a dramatic clinical symptomatic improvement with the use of 5 g of 2% clindamycin cream administered daily for 4–6 weeks with an initial clinical improvement in more than 90% of the patients. However, a high relapse rate was also reported. In a further follow-up study published in 2011, in which more than 100 women were followed, the relapse rate varied from 25 to 35% on cessation of 4 weeks of clindamycin therapy. Women experiencing high relapse, however, responded to the reintroduction of clindamycin therapy, which was then given on a maintenance basis, using a reduced volume and a more infrequent basis. Thus the chronicity of the clinical syndrome was appreciated together with the need to recommend therapy for months, if not years, in order to control if not cure the patients. Long-term cure rates remain unknown, although the overwhelming majority of the patients are readily controlled. Experience with intravaginal 10% hydrocortisone, which unfortunately is not available commercially, or with clobetasol gel, had similarly resulted in excellent early response rates, but no evidence has emerged of superiority over topical clindamycin. Both regimens represent off-label use of medications, including the need to have the cortisone prepared by compounding pharmacies. Patients should be followed on a regular basis as the dose of the intravaginal therapy is titrated downward. Incomplete clinical response should prompt consideration of adding topical estrogen therapy due to frequent unrecognized estrogen deficiency. Also, vulvar and vestibular inflammation may occasionally merit additional topical steroid therapy.

Bibliography

Berg, AO, Heidrich, FE, Fihn, SD, et al. Establishing the cause of genitourinary symptoms in women in a family practice: Comparison of clinical examination and comprehensive microbiology. *J Am Med Assoc* 1984; **251**: 620.

Donders G, Bellen G, Byttebier G, et al. Individualized decreasing-dose maintenance fluconazole regimen for recurrent vulvovaginal candidiasis (ReCiDiF trial). *Am J Obstet Gynecol* 2008 Dec; 199 (6):613. e1–9.

Donders GG, Babula O, Bellen G, et al. Mannose-binding lectin gene polymorphism and resistance to therapy in women with recurrent vulvovaginal candidiasis. *Br J Gynecol* 2008; **115** (10):1225–1231.

Duerr, A, Helig, CM, Meikle, SF, et al. Incident and persistent vulvovaginal candidiasis among human immunodeficiency virus-infected women: Risk factors and severity. *Obstet Gynecol* 2003; **101**: 548.

Eckert LO. Clinical practice. Acute vulvovaginitis. *New Engl J Med* 2006; **355**: 1244–1252.

Ferwerda B, Ferwerda G, Plantinga TS, et al. Human dectin-1 deficiency and mucocutaneous fungal infections. *New Engl J Med* 2009; **361**: 1760–1767.

Fleury, FJ. Adult vaginitis. *Clin Obstet Gynecol* 1981; **24**: 407.

Giraldo, PC, Babula, O, Goncalves, AK, et al. Mannose-Binding Lectin Gene Polymorphism, Vulvovaginal Candidiasis, and Bacterial Vaginosis. *Obstet Gynecol* 2007; **109**: 1123.

Messinger-Rapport BJ, Thacker HL. Prevention for the older woman. A practical guide to hormone replacement therapy and urogynecologic health. *Geriatrics* 2001; **56**: 32-34, 37-38 40–42.

Netea MG, Brown GD, Kullberg BJ, Gow NA. An integrated model of the recognition of Candida albicans by the innate immune system. *Nat Rev Microbiol* 2008; **6**: 67–78.

North American Menopause Society. The role of local vaginal estrogen for treatment of vaginal atrophy in postmenopausal women: 2007 position statement of The North American Menopause Society. *Menopause* 2007; **14**: 355–369

Nyirjesy P, Peyton C, Weitz MV, et al. Causes of chronic vaginitis: analysis of a prospective database of affected women. *Obstet Gynecol* 2006; **108**: 1185–1191.

Pappas PG, Kauffman CA, Andes D, et al. Clinical practice guidelines for the management of candidiasis: 2009 update by the Infectious Diseases Society of America. *Clin Infect Dis* 2009; **48**: 503–535.

Patel DA, Gillespie B, Sobel JD, et al. Risk factors for recurrent vulvovaginal candidiasis in women receiving maintenance antifungal therapy: results of a prospective cohort study. *Am J Obstet Gynecol* 2004; **190**: 644–653.

Pirotta, M, Gunn, J, Chondros, P, et al. Effect of lactobacillus in preventing post-antibiotic vulvovaginal candidiasis: a randomised controlled trial. *Br Med J* 2004; **329**: 548.

Ray D, Goswami R, Banerjee U, et al. Prevalence of Candida glabrata and its response to boric acid vaginal suppositories in comparison with oral fluconazole in patients with diabetes and vulvovaginal candidiasis. *Diabetes Care* 2007; **30**: 312–317.

Sobel JD. Desquamative inflammatory vaginitis: a new subgroup of purulent vaginitis responsive to topical 2% clindamycin therapy. *Am J Obstet Gynecol* 1994; **171**: 1215–1220.

Sobel JD. Non-trichomonal Purulent Vaginitis: Clinical Approach. *Curr Infect Dis Rep* 2000; **2**: 501–505.

Sobel JD, Chaim W. Treatment of Torulopsis glabrata vaginitis: retrospective review of boric acid therapy. *Clin Infect Dis* 1997; **24**: 649–652.

Sobel JD. *Management of patients with recurrent vulvovaginal candidiasis*. Drugs 2003; **63**: 1059.

Sobel JD, Wiesenfeld HC, Martens M, et al. Maintenance fluconazole therapy for recurrent vulvovaginal candidiasis. *New Engl J Med* 2004; **351**: 876.

Sobel JD. Vulvovaginal candidosis. *Lancet* 2007; **369**: 1961–1971.

Sobel JD, Reichman O, Misra D, Yoo W. Prognosis and treatment of desquamative inflammatory vaginitis. *Obstet Gynecol* 2011; **117**: 850–855.

Stockdale CK. Clinical spectrum of desquamative inflammatory vaginitis. *Curr Infect Dis Rep* 2010; **12**: 479–483.

Tabrizi SN, Pirotta MV, Rudland E, Garland SM. Detection of Candida species by PCR in self-collected vaginal swabs of women after taking antibiotics. *Mycoses* 2006; **49**: 523–524.

Human Papillomavirus

Suzanne M. Garland

Department of Microbiology and Infectious Diseases, The Royal Women's Hospital, Department of Obstetrics and Gynaecology, University of Melbourne, and Murdoch Children's Research Institute, Parkville, Victoria, Australia

HPV the virus

Human papillomaviruses (HPVs) belong to a large family of heterogeneous viruses (Papillomavirideae), which are species specific. They are small double-stranded DNA viruses that specifically infect squamous and mucosal epithelia. These viruses are not efficiently propagated by traditional viral culture techniques because the viral life cycle of HPVs is intimately linked to the maturation of squamous epithelium and thus complete virion production only occurs in the terminally differentiated squamous epithelial cells. The complete cycle, from initial infection of the basal cell to expression of fully infectious viruses in shed fully differentiated epithelium, takes in the order of 2 to 3 weeks. With this complexity, the detection of HPV has relied on molecular technologies which, when applied in good epidemiological studies, has determined that cervical cancer is the first cancer to be caused, virtually 100%, by a virus. There are almost 130 HPV genotypes identified largely by the sequencing of the gene encoding the major capsid protein L1. Of the large number of HPVs, there is tropism for infection for different tissues by various genotypes; i.e. skin types (e.g. HPV 1–4, 10, 26–29, 37, 38, 46, 47, 49, 50, 57), and genital types for which there around 30–40 (e.g. HPV 6, 11, 16, 18, various 30s, 40s, 50s, 60s, 70s). The genital types are divided into those with a high oncogenic potential, particularly HPV 16, 18, 30s (31, 33, 35, 39), 45, 50s (52, 54, 56, 58, 59) and 60s (68) possible (HPV 26, 53, 66, 67, 73, 82), or low risk (6, 11, 40, 42, 43, 44, 54, 70).

HPV oncogenic potential for cervical disease

HPV 16 and 18 behave as more virulent viruses, causing a greater proportion of cervical disease (~50% and 20% respectively of cancers), causing disease earlier, as well as being more likely to persist than other high-risk HPV types. Of note, worldwide types 16 and 18 contribute to ~70% of all squamous cell cervical cancers and around 80% for adenocarcinoma. In molecular epidemiological studies (case control studies) it has been shown that the strength of association for HPV 16/18 is very strong with odds ratios (ORs) several hundred-fold, being far greater than the 10-fold association of smoking and lung cancer. After these two types, the next most common types contribute a smaller proportion individually. For example, globally HPV 33, 45, and 31 are the third, fourth, and fifth most common types respectively, and collectively they account for an additional ~10% of cervical cancer cases. There are some variations geographically: for example,

---

Sexually Transmitted Diseases, First Edition. Edited by Richard H. Beigi.

in Asia, types 58, 33, and 52 are seen more prominently after 16 and 18 than elsewhere. When specifically looking at adenocarcinomas – a cancer that eludes detection by cytology screening – it is noteworthy that HPV 18 plays a greater role than it does for squamous cell cancers. HPV 18, 16, and 45 are the first, second, and third most common types respectively, collectively accounting for almost 90% of all cases. In addition to cervical cancer, HPV 16 and 18 collectively cause 50% of high-grade pre-cancerous lesions (cervical intraepithelial neoplasia [CIN] grade 2/3 both squamous cell and adenocarcinoma ACIS) and around one quarter (~13 to 25%) of low-grade CIN (CIN 1).

Cofactors

Recognized cofactors that act in conjunction with oncogenic HPV infection to increase the risk of invasive cervical cancer include: cigarette smoking, younger age at first intercourse, high parity, long-term use of oral contraceptive pill, and other sexually transmitted infections (e.g. *Chlamydia trachomatis,* anogenital herpes simplex). However, in general, each of these factors has ORs in the order of 2 or less, and some could be confounded by sexual behavior.

Epidemiology

Cervical cancer is the second most common cancer of women world wide. The brunt of the burden is borne by the developing world largely due to the lack of effective screening programs to detect and treat pre-cancerous lesions. Overall incidence is in the order of half a million cases annually with around a quarter of a million deaths per annum world wide. It is to be noted that cervical cancer occurs in relatively young women, around 40 to 50 years – an age when many women are still significantly contributing to their family upbringing.

HPV oncogenic potential noncervical disease

Oncogenic HPVs are also strongly linked to a subset of other female anogenital cancers, specifically vulvar, vaginal, and anal cancers, with HPV being associated in approximately 40, 40, and 90% respectively.

In males, HPV-related anogenital cancers include anal and penile, of which approximately 90% and 50%, respectively, are HPV related. In addition to anogenital cancers, oncogenic HPV types (particularly type 16) have been linked to a proportion (~ 15–25%) of oropharyngeal cancers. Globally, approximately 4% of all cancers are associated with HPV.

Low-risk HPV-related disease: genital warts

Low-risk HPV types cause a proportion of low-grade cervical lesions as well as benign, hyperproliferative lesions commonly referred to as genital warts (or condylomata acuminata). Genital warts (GWs) are the most common viral sexually transmitted disease, being caused by HPV types 6 and 11 in around 90% of cases. The prevalence typically peaks in mid-twenties; infectivity is high, with two-thirds of sexual partners complaining of warts. The time from HPV infection to GW development is as short as 2–3 months. It is noteworthy that the incidence of GWs has been increasing over the past few decades. The main indication for treatment of GWs is alleviation of symptoms (pruritis, bleeding, burning, tenderness), or for psychosocial distress. Untreated, GWs may resolve spontaneously, increase in size and number, or remain unchanged. Treatment is crude, being largely destructive (cryotherapy, electrocautery, laser, surgery) chemotoxic, or immunomodulatory with imiquimod. The choice is largely guided by patient preference, number of lesions, anatomical site, as well as cost. There is no definitive evidence suggesting that one treatment is superior to others. The treatment regimens are either patient-applied or physician-applied. As all of the regiments have shortcomings, some clinicians use combination therapy.

Patient-applied medications include:

(a) Podophyllotoxin 0.15% cream or 0.5% paint topically applied to each wart, twice daily for 3 days followed by a 4-day break, then repeat weekly for up to 4 cycles or until the warts disappear. Podophyllotoxin, although cheap and relatively easy to use, is an antimytotic and should not be used in pregnancy. It is recommended that the first application should be made by the clinician to demonstrate the appropriate method. Irritation or mild to moderate pain may follow.

(b) Another patient-applied alternative is imiquimod 5% cream – an immune enhancing modulator which stimulates the production of interferon and other cytokines. It is approved for the treatment of external GWs but not for vaginal, cervical, or urethral administration. The cream should be applied once daily at bedtime, three times per week. The treatment area needs to be washed off 6–10 hours after application. Local inflammatory reactions such as redness, irritation, and vesiculation may be seen, while some common hypopigmentation can occur. It is noteworthy that imiquimod might weaken condoms and vaginal diaphragms, and the safety of imiquimod during pregnancy has not been established.

(c) Another alternative is sinecatechins 15% ointment, a green-tea extract with an active product (catechins). This should be applied three times daily using a finger to ensure coverage with a thin layer of ointment until the complete clearance of warts. This product should not be continued for longer than 16 weeks, and does not need washing off after application.

Provider-administered regimens include:

(a) Cryotherapy with liquid nitrogen or cryoprobe. Repeat applications every 1–2 weeks. Cryotherapy is destructive by thermal-induced cytolysis. This can be painful and followed by necrosis and not infrequently by blistering.

(b) Trichloroacetic acid (TCA) 80%–90%. TCA is a caustic agent and the biochemical coagulation of proteins destroys the GWs. Due to its low viscosity, one needs to be careful in its application to ensure that it does not run on to normal adjacent skin. Ensure that it has dried before the patient leaves. This treatment can be applied weekly as necessary.

(c) Surgical removal, either by tangential scissor excision, tangential shave excision, curettage, electrosurgery, or carbon dioxide laser. This is largely reserved for a large number of GWs, all particularly in other anatomical sites such as urethral, but requires surgical expertise.

In general, treatment can be painful and often results in considerable patient dissatisfaction due to the relatively high recurrence rates. This should be thoroughly discussed with patients before embarking on therapy. In addition, genital warts can also cause psychosocial distress, similar to that seen for high grade dysplasia. They also carry a high financial burden.

Recurrent respiratory laryngeal papillomatosis

RRP is a rare disease occurring at an incidence of 0.3–1.0/100 000, with pediatric as well as adult onset types. They carry significant morbidity and mortality and are largely attributable to HPV types 6 and 11. For the juvenile onset type (JORRP), HPV is thought to be transmitted vertically from mother to child during the birth process. In around a third of children with JORRP, lesions spread into the trachea and bronchi with the risk of respiratory obstruction.

Natural history of HPV infection

Women

Overall, genital HPV infections (as determined by HPV DNA detection) are extremely common. In fact most sexually active individuals (around 60–80%) will become infected at some stage over their lifetime. Moreover most genital HPV infections are acquired sexually, with infection occurring shortly after onset of first sexual debut. It may also be transmitted by intimate contact: genital-to-genital skin contact without penetrative sexual intercourse. Therefore it is important in discussing HPV infection with patients that the commonality of infection is realized, that HPV is not like traditional sexually transmitted infections and therefore should be destigmatized. Most HPV infections are transient (HPV DNA can no longer be detected when using highly sensitive assays such as polymerase chain reaction [PCR]), while a small proportion become chronic or persistent (same genotype positive at least 6 months apart).

With the commonality of this infection, high transmissibility, in women the curves of prevalence typically show a sharp rise after sexual debut, peaking around 25 years, then slowly declining to a level of around five to 10% in those over 30 years of age. Globally, the prevalence of

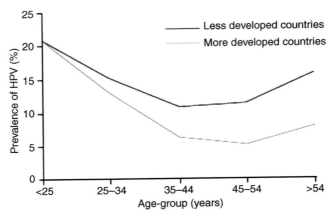

Figure 10.1. World estimates on the age-specific HPV prevalence by country-specific development status. Age-specific HPV prevalence estimates derived from the meta-analysis applied to the female population within each 10-year age group by development area. Countries were classified as less or more developed, according to Globocan. (Reproduced from De Sanjose, et al. *Lancet Infectious Diseases* 2007; **7:** 453–459, with permission from Elsevier.)

HPV overall in a large meta-analysis of almost 160,000 women with normal cytology was estimated at just over 10%. Figures 10.1 and 10.2 respectively show the variability in age specific prevalence patterns in women from developing and developed different regions of the world, plus regional variabilities. It can be seen that in some populations a second smaller peak is seen in those 40 year old plus. Various explanations for this include changes in sexual behaviour, cohort effect, or with the relative immune senescence of ageing reflection of reactivation of latent infection.

It is noteworthy that HPV can also be transmitted from mother to child during birth: consequently a young child with genital warts may have contracted infection from the mother and not necessarily intimate sexual abuse. Such cases need careful evaluation by those specialized in the area. Such transmission from mother to child can also result uncommonly in RRP.

Genital warts can certainly grown extensively in pregnancy and be very difficult to manage due to the high recurrence rate until pregnancy has been completed. Regimens which are safe in pregnancy include cryotherapy and surgery. Due to the

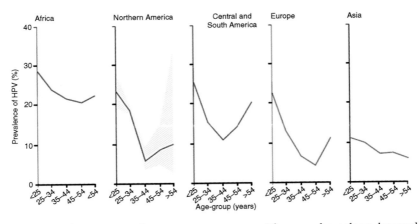

Figure 10.2. Age-specific HPV prevalence among women with normal cytology, by world region. Shaded areas represent 95% CIs. (Reproduced from De Sanjose, et al. *Lancet Infectious Diseases* 2007; **7:** 453–459, with permission from Elsevier.)

large bulk, GW may cause pelvic outlet obstruction and require Caesarean delivery. Caesarean section however is not recommended to prevent HPV transmission in order to prevent RRP.

Clearance of most infection occurs within a short period of time, the majority resolving within 12 months. However, in the small proportion (10–20%) in whom HPV remains chronic (the determinants of persistence and progression are not fully understood, but are likely to be genetic and/or environmental factors), women are at risk of developing cellular abnormalities of high-grade dysplasia, the obligate precursor of cancer.

Males

In contrast to women, the natural history of HPV in males is largely unknown. In several prevalence surveys in males in contrast to that of women, prevalence shows a flat line (Figure 10.3). What this actually means is yet to be determined. In a recent cohort study of just over 1,100 healthy men, incidence of a new genital HPV infection was reported at 38.4 per 1,000 person months. Not surprisingly oncogenic HPV infection was significantly associated with a higher number of lifetime female sexual partners, number of male anal-sex partners. Median duration of HPV infection was 7.5 months for any HPV and 12 months for HPV 16. Clearance of HPV decreased in those men with a higher number of lifetime partners.

Latent HPV infection

A small proportion of HPV-infected individuals are likely to have latent infection (ie the virus can remain within basal epithelial cells either arrested or very slowly replicating, but undetectable by current DNA technology). Such latent infections may become reactivated, particularly in the circumstance of immune senescence or immune-suppression. The extent to which latency occurs is currently unknown, but may well explain exacerbation of cervical pre-cancerous

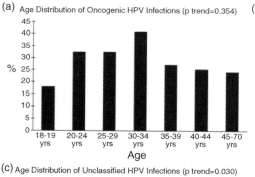

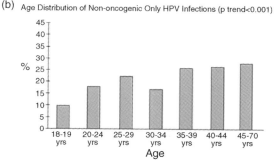

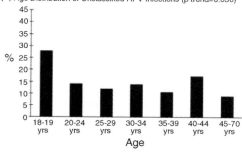

Figure 10.3. HPV prevalence at enrolment by age: **A,** any oncogenic HPV infection; **B,** nononcogenic HPV infection only; **C,** unclassified infections. (Adapted and reprinted by permission from the American Association for Cancer Research: Anna R. Giuliano, Eduardo Lazcano-Ponce, Luisa L. Villa, et al., The human papillomavirus infection in men study: human papillomavirus prevalence and type distribution among men residing in Brazil, Mexico, and the United States. *Cancer Epidemiol Biomarkers Prev* 2008; **17:** 2036–2043.)

lesions or genital warts, particularly among women with defective cell-mediated immunity or as seen with aging, yet with no reinfection or new exposure to HPV infection. Therefore, in counseling a couple who are adamant that there has been mutual monogamy for years, it should be recognized and discussed that latency may well be an explanation for a new dysplastic lesion.

> ⚠ **CAUTION!**
>
> - Genital HPV is a very common infection transmitted predominantly by sexual contact, with most infections being transient.
> - It is so common that it should not be treated as a traditional STI per se when counseling patients, but rather be destigmatized.

Cervical cytology manifestations of HPV

It is now recognized that CIN 1 represents the cytopathic effect of HPV viral infection in tissue and not necessarily the beginning of the progression to cancer as was once believed. CIN 1 is caused by both high- and low-risk HPVs, and usually transient, resolving with the development of a host cell-mediated immune response. HPV in CIN 1 lesions is maintained in an episomal form, with complete viral replication and infectious virus shed from the terminal epithelium. In contrast high-grade lesions or CIN 2/3 are largely caused by high-risk HPVs, and there is dysregulation, particularly of the E 6/E7 genes and incomplete viral replication. In CIN 3, there is full thickness involvement of the epithelium with the histological features of genetically unstable lesions being noted with aneuploidy. In some cases the HPV becomes incorporated into the host genome as integrated HPV.

Cin 3: The True Precursor Lesion to Cervical Cancer

It is now accepted that CIN 2 or CIN 3 can occur *de novo*, rather than result as a continuum from CIN 1 lesions. In fact, the true precursor lesion to cancer is CIN 3, with many now realizing that CIN 2 cases are a mixed group of low-grade and true high-grade lesions. CIN 3 lesions, if untreated, will have a progression rate to cancer of ~30–40%, and consequently, are always recommended for treatment. They are largely due to high-risk HPVs. Determining which will regress and which will progress, has led to the study of other biomarkers for progression, although none is yet ready at the diagnostic level, and cannot yet guide the definite need for certain CIN 3 lesions to be treated. It should also be noted that the majority of CIN 3 and cancers occur around the transformation zone (TZ) of the cervix; adequate ablation of the precursor lesions and the TZ effectively prevents development of cervical cancers.

Persistent oncogenic HPV infection precedes CIN 3

In a small proportion of women, infection remains persistent, remaining unchanged for years. It is persistent infection with an oncogenic virus which puts a woman at risk for development of CIN 3. Moreover, it has been shown by several groups that those infected with high-risk (HR) HPV (as measured by Hybrid Capture 2 test [HC2]) at baseline, and with a normal Pap who were followed over 10 years, had a risk of cytologic abnormality of atypical squamous abnormalities or worse. At 5 years the rate is around 20% and for CIN 2+ it is 10%.

Looking at the 10-year positive predictive value of a single positive HR HPV DNA for cytological prediction of CIN 3+ it is around 20%. When evaluating outcome for those with two HR HPV tests at 5 and 10 years, this risk increases from around 9% to 20% respectively. Of particular note has been the value of a concurrent high-risk HPV negative test in cytologically normal women: this therefore carries a high long-term negative predictive value being > 99% for CIN 2+ and CIN 3+, suggesting that the screening interval might be safely increased. For this reason, some are advocating the use of HPV DNA testing with Pap cytology for screening. When looking specifically at HPV specific genotypes, detecting and differentiating HPV 16 and 18 infections from the other potentially oncogenic types may better identify women at risk for developing CIN 3.

Prevention of cervical cancer by screening for and treating pre-neoplastic lesions

In those countries where effective high coverage of high-quality cervical cytology screening programs are maintained, which not only target the appropriate population but result in treatment and adequate follow-up, incidence as well as mortality from cervical cancer falls significantly. Good cervical cytology screening programs come not only at a high cost monetarily, but also in infrastructure as well as the maintenance of well-trained high-quality cytotechnicians. Where programs are opportunistic, have poor coverage, and lack quality control measures, minimal impact is seen. Therefore, for resource-poor countries, other screening methods with reduced costs have been evaluated; for example, visual inspection with acidic acid (VIA) has been assessed but also requires good training staff to "see and treat" aceto-white areas. More recently rapid HPV DNA assays have been evaluated and look very promising, being more objective in determining underlying lesions for treatment.

Immunology

The host immune response from natural HPV infection involves both humoral and cell-mediated compartments. However, the humoral antibody response occurs slowly and is generally weak. Only around 50–60% of individuals who are HPV DNA positive mount a measurable antibody response. Despite this finding in humans, animal studies show that neutralizing antibodies from primary papillomavirus infections are protective. It should be noted that an antibody response is largely type specific. Thus it is thought that there is some natural immunity from infection, although it is probably incomplete. This is based on looking at genotype sequences of individuals infected initially with HPV who, when followed longitudinally with intermittently positive tests, show the same HPV sequence, suggesting reactivation from the original infection and rather than reinfection per se. Clearance of HPV infection and resolution of clinical lesions such as genital warts is characterized by an effective cell mediated immune response.

It should also be noted that various serological assays have been used in sero-epidemiological studies as well as in vaccine trials. They are not recommended for use clinically for diagnosis.

Prophylactic HPV vaccines

Two first-generation prophylactic HPV vaccines have been licensed to date and both are subunit protein vaccines. They utilize recombinant DNA technology, whereby the HPV late protein gene (L1) which encodes for the outer viral capsid is expressed in a vector such as eukaryotic cells (*Saccromyces cerevisiae* yeast cells or *Spodoptera frugiperda* (Sf9) ovarian cells, the natural host for baculovirus). These empty capsid VLPs self-assemble into so-called "virus-like particles" (VLPs) and effectively mimic a natural HPV viral infection, but are not infectious, given that they do not contain any DNA. The vaccines are different in that the quadrivalent vaccine Gardasil® consists of HPV 6, 11, 16, and 18 L1 VLPs plus an aluminum hydroxyphosphate sulfate adjuvant. The bivalent vaccine known as Cervarix® consists of HPV 16 and 18 L1 VLPs adjuvanted with an aluminum hydroxide–monophosphoryl lipid A complex, ASO4.

Efficacy

The quadrivalent human papillomavirus (HPV 6, 11, 16, 18) vaccine and the bivalent vaccine (HPV 16, 18) have been licensed for use in clinical practice since June 2006 and May 2007, respectively. Licensure was largely based on phase 3 clinical trials which showed high efficacy against disease for the vaccine-related strains covered by the respective vaccines, high immunogenicity elicited, as well as excellent safety profiles. Specifically, for the quadrivalent vaccine, phase 3 clinical trials in women 16–26 years have shown near 100% efficacy against HPV 16- and/or 18-related precursor lesions to cervical, vulvar, and vaginal cancers; i.e. cervical, vulvar, and vaginal intraepithelial neoplasias grades 2/3 (CIN 2/3, VIN 2/3, VaIN 2/3) respectively, for those naïve to HPV 16 and/or 18.

More recently similar phase 3 clinical trials in men 16–26 years have shown high efficacy (~90%) against HPV 6-, 11-,16-, and/or 18-related external genital lesions, including the precursor lesions anal intraepithelial neoplasia (AIN 2/3, as a surrogate for anal cancer), as well as penile intraepithelial neoplasia (PIN 2/3, as a surrogate for penile cancer). Near 100% prophylactic efficacy has also been shown against HPV 6- and 11-related genital warts for both males and females.

Phase 3 placebo-controlled clinical trials for the quadrivalent (HPV 6, 11, 16, 18) vaccine have been reported for almost 20,000 young women and girls, plus just over 4,000 young men and boys aged 16–26 years from around 20 countries and showed high immunogenicity, excellent safety, and efficacy against external genital warts for both genders, as well as high-grade intraepithelial lesions at the cervix, vagina, and vulva in women, and anus in males, in those naive to HPV 6, 11, 16 and/or 18 at baseline.

Specifically for the bivalent vaccine, in the final analysis (mean follow-up of 35 months) very high efficacy for protection from infection (80% and 76% protection against HPV 16 or 18 for six months and 12 months respectively), and for high-grade cervical dysplasia (93%) for those naïve to HPV 16 and/or 18 (by both HPV DNA and serology) at baseline has been shown. A type assignment analysis was performed to assign probable causality: efficacy for CIN 2+ for 16/18 in those naive at baseline was 98%. More extensive follow-up data is forthcoming.

• Phase 3 placebo-controlled clinical trials for the bivalent (HPV 16, 18) vaccine have been reported for almost 20,000 young women and girls, ages 16-26 years from around 14 countries from four global regions (North America, Latin America, Europe and Asia-Pacific) and showed high immunogenicity, excellent safety, and efficacy against high-grade intraepithelial lesions at the cervix, for those naïve to HPV 16 and/or 18 at baseline.

Both vaccines show some cross-protection for infection and disease for HPV genotypes phylogenetically related to 16 and 18. For the quadrivalent vaccine this is largely driven by protection against HPV 31, whereas for the bivalent vaccine there was significant protection against persistent infection (6 months) for 31 (79%), 33 (46%), and HPV 45 (76%), and for 12 months infection [against HPV 31 (79%), HPV 33 (38%), HPV 45 (63%) This cross-protection extended to significant protection for disease for HPV 31 CIN 2+ (92%), as well as for CIN 2+ for 12 combined oncogenic types not including 16 or 18 at 54%. It is noteworthy that there was a statistically significant reduction in colposcopy referrals (10%), as well as ablative cervical procedures (25%) in those vaccinated.

The durability and clinical significance of this cross-protection will be realized by long-term follow-up of vaccine recipients.

Safety

Injection site pain, redness, and swelling were significantly more frequent among subjects receiving either quadrivalent or the bivalent vaccine than placebo or the hepatitis A vaccine respectively. The safety profile otherwise for those vaccinated with the either vaccine is high. Estimated rates of urticaria or syncope (alone) for the quadrivalent vaccine are in the order of 78 cases per million doses, syncope with seizures 28 cases per million doses and anaphylaxis 7.8 cases per million doses.

• Prophylactic HPV vaccines are not recommended for use in pregnancy. However, should a woman inadvertently be vaccinated when pregnant, this is not an indication for termination of pregnancy. The vaccines are subunit, not live, have no DNA and in follow-up of inadvertent use in pregnancy have not shown any increased adverse outcome.

Vaccine effectiveness in real life scenarios

In real life settings where the quadrivalent vaccine is being used with high population coverage (schoolgirls 11–12 years with catch up to 26), significant reductions are being seen already in those diseases with the shortest incubation period: i.e. reductions in genital warts is reported (for this age group in females, plus in males from herd immunity), as well as for high-grade cervical cytology abnormalities in young women. Similar data is expected soon for the bivalent vaccine.

For those with past infection with clearance of HPV DNA (serologically positive, but HPV DNA negative) there is evidence that this subgroup, when vaccinated with either quadrivalent or bivalent vaccine, are protected from ongoing lesions due to the vaccine-related type to which they were previously naturally infected.

Target populations

As both the bivalent and quadrivalent HPV vaccines are prophylactic, the greatest impact in the prevention of vaccine-related-HPV infection and disease is the administration of the vaccines to sexually inexperienced young girls and/or boys.

Sexually experienced populations

Both vaccines show efficacy, safety, and immunogenicity in adult women, who are already sexually active. However, the gain is not as great as it is for those who have not been infected previously; consequently the primary target for vaccination is young girls prior to sexual debut.

Moreover, as both vaccines are prophylactic and not therapeutic, those with prevalent infections or disease prior to, or at the time of, vaccination only gain protection for those types to which they have not been previously infected. However, a young woman who is currently infected with HPV 16, but not HPV 6, 11 or 18 (in the case of the quadrivalent) or not with HPV 18 (in the case of the bivalent), will gain protection for HPV 6, 11, and 18, but not for 16 (in the case of the quadrivalent vaccine). She will gain protection for 18 (in the case of the bivalent vaccine), but not for 16 equally as well if she were completely naive for all four or two types respectively.

Moreover, in sexually active young women who have been vaccinated (with either vaccine) and treated for cervical lesions subsequently (and for the quadrivalent vaccine, those treated for external genital warts) there is a significant reduction in ongoing incident lesions as compared to those nonvaccinated.

★ **TIPS & TRICKS**

Even though sexually active individuals can gain protection from infection and/or disease from which they have not yet been infected, there is no routine serological assay used diagnostically to screen individuals for past exposure. Moreover, at a public health level, is not recommended to screen individuals for the presence of HPV DNA as this would not define whether a particular individual has been previously, currently, transiently, or persistently infected.

Challenges

Current schedules for vaccination require intramuscular injections of three doses spread over 6 months. Ongoing research is examining the impact of different schedules as well as the efficacy of two-dose regimens. The biggest challenges currently are: to ensure affordable prices for these effective vaccines to be endorsed by governments and policymakers, and to ensure appropriate coverage to translate into a real reduction in disease – particularly for those countries with the greatest burden of disease.

✋ **CAUTION!**

- Even though vaccine efficacy against HPV 16- and 18-related disease is extremely high, these types contribute to ∼70% of high-grade cervical disease; consequently, all females who have been vaccinated (whether as schoolgirls or as sexually active adult women) must be actively encouraged to continue cervical cytology screening for cervical lesions.

Vulvar and vaginal cancers

Vulvar cancer is a less common disease to that of the cervix, with global incidence rates ranging from 0.1 to 3.5 per 100,000 women for the years 1998–2002. Nonetheless, vulval and vaginal cancer collectively account for approximately 6% of all gynecological cancers. In contrast to secondary cancer prevention programs for cervical cancers, no such programs exist for vaginal and vulval malignancies. The annual progression rate of untreated vulvar intraepithelial neoplasia (VIN 3) to invasive cancer is at least 10%, whereas for CIN 3 to cancer is approximately 2%. Patients with vaginal intraepithelial neoplasia (VaIN) have a 2% risk of developing invasive cancer. Diagnosis of VIN and VaIN is difficult, as is their treatment which can be disfiguring and requires very long-term follow-up, as disease recurrence is common. Due to the multifocal nature of HPV, those with cervical disease are more likely to have HPV-related VIN and/or VaIN; the corollary is also true.

Anal cancer

Oncogenic HPVs have also been linked to around 90% of anal cancers. In evaluating the age-adjusted incidence rates of primary anal cancers by gender and year of diagnosis, there has been a steady increase in the rates for males, as well as females, in the past four decades.

Given the greater risk and incidence of anal cancer, and the recognition of progression of high-grade anal intraepithelial neoplasia (AIN 2/3) to anal squamous cell carcinoma in HIV-positive men who have sex with men (MSM), it is proposed by some clinicians to screen for AIN in HIV-positive MSM and possibly HIV-positive women (and possibly those with other immunocompromised states such as transplant recipients) using anal cytology, high-resolution anoscopy (HRA), with directed HRA biopsy for definitive diagnosis. Implementing such screening strategies requires cytologists trained in anal cytology, clinicians trained in HRA, as well as appropriate treatment and follow-up of AIN 2/3. In addition, while some recommend ablating AIN 2/3 when it is diagnosed, others keep it under careful surveillance. As there are divergent views with respect to screening for and management of AIN 2/3, appropriate guidelines for care are required.

Penile cancer

Oncogenic HPVs have also been linked to around 40% of penile cancers, which is quite rare and constitutes less than 1% of all male cancers. Incidence rates are recorded in the order of 1 per 100,000. HPV is associated with a proportion of the pre-cancerous high-grade dysplastic lesions of penile intraepithelial neoplasias (PIN).

Oropharyngeal cancer

Oncogenic HPVs have also been linked to around 15–25% of oropharyngeal cancers, most notably tonsillar, with reports up to 70% positive for HPV16. Again, as with vulvar cancer, epidemiology suggests two distinct types: (1) those in older individuals associated with smoking and alcohol intake and not related to HPV, whereas (2) the HPV-related cancers are in younger individuals with no association with the aforementioned cofactors, and have a better prognosis overall. While the former have not changed in incidence, the HPV-related oropharyngeal cancers are increasing. In studies looking at the oral carriage of HPV, the prevalence has been reported at around 10%.

Bibliography

Agorastos T, Chatzigeorgiou K, Brotherton JM, et al. Safety of human papillomavirus (HPV) vaccines: a review of the international experience so far. *Vaccine* 2009; **27**(52): 7270–7281.

Belinson S, Smith, J.S., Myers E, et al. Risk factors for cervical intra-epithelial neoplasia grade 2 appear more similar to grade 1 than grade 3. *Cancer Epidemiol Biom Preven* 2008 Sep; **17**(9): 2350–2355.

Brotherton JML, Fridman M, May CL, et al. Early effect of the HPV vaccination programme on cervical abnormalities in Victoria, Australia: an ecological study. *Lancet* 2011; **377**: 2085–2092.

De Sanjose S, Quint WGV, Alemany L, et al. (On behalf of the RIS HPV TT Study Group.) Human papillomavirus genotype attribution in invasive cervical cancer: a retrospective cross-sectional worldwide study. *Lancet Oncol* 2010; **11**: 1048–1056.

Donovan B, Franklin N, Guy R, et al. Quadrivalent human papillomavirus vaccination and trends in genital warts in Australia: analysis of national sentinel surveillance data. *Lancet* 2010; **11**(1): 39–44.

Fox P. Anal cancer screening in men who have sex with men. *Curr Opin HIV AIDS* 2009; **4**: 64–67.

Garland SM, Steben M, Sings H, et al. Natural history of genital warts: analysis of the placebo arm of two randomized phase 3 trials of a quadrivalent HPV (types 6, 11, 16, 18) vaccine. *J Infect Dis* 2009. Mar; **199**(6): 805–814.

Giuliano AR, Lee JH, Fulp W, Villa LL, Lazcano E, et al. Incidence and clearance of genital human papillomavirus infection in men (HIM): a cohort study. *Lancet.* 2011 Mar; **377**(9769): 932–940.

Hagensee ME, Yaegashi NM, Galloway DA. Self-assembly of human papillomavirus type 1 capsids by expression of the L1 protein alone or by coexpression of the L1 and L2 capsid proteins. *J Virol* 1993; **67**(1): 315–322.

Munk C, Nielsen A, Kjaer S (eds.). Penile cancer – incidence in Danish men 1978–2003. The 25th International Papillomavirus Conference, Malmö, Sweden, 2009.

Paavonen J, Naud P, Salmeron J, et al. (for the HPV, PATRICIA, Study, Group). Efficacy of human papillomavirus (HPV)-16/18 AS04-adjuvanted vaccine against cervical infection and precancer caused by oncogenic HPV types (PATRICIA): final analysis of a double-blind, randomised study in young women. *Lancet* 2009; **374**: 301–314.

Palefsky JM. Anal cancer prevention in HIV-positive men and women. *Curr Opin Oncol* 2009; **21**: 433–438.

Rose RC, et al. Expression of human papillomavirus type 11 L1 protein in insect cells: in vivo and in vitro assembly of viruslike particles. *J Virol* 1993; **67**(4): 1936–1944.

Stanley M. Review: Potential mechanisms for HPV vaccine-induced long-term protection. *Gynecol Oncol* 2010; **118**: S2–S7.

Smith JS, Lindsay LJ, Hoots B, et al. Human papillomavirus type distribution in invasive cervical cancer and high-grade cervical lesions: a meta-analysis update. *Int J Cancer* 2007; **121**(3): 621–632.

Wallboomers JM, Jacobs MV, Manos MM, et al. Human papillomavirus is a necessary cause of invasive cervical cancer worldwide. *J Pathol* 1999; **189**: 12–19.

Ectoparasites: Pediculosis Pubis and Scabies

Amber Naresh and Richard H. Beigi

Department of Obstetrics, Gynecology and Reproductive Sciences, Division of Reproductive Infectious Diseases, Magee-Womens Hospital of the University of Pittsburgh Medical Center, Pittsburgh, PA, USA

Pediculosis pubis

Background

Pediculosis pubis, commonly called pubic lice, is caused by the crab louse, *Phthrirus pubis*. The organism is 1 to 2 mm long, yellow-gray, and square-shaped. Its six legs end in a claw adapted for clasping hairs. It is smaller and squat in appearance compared to the human body or head louse (Figure 11.1).

Crab lice prefer pubic, axillary, and body hair, although rarely, beard, scalp, eyebrow, and eyelash infestations may occur. This likely has to do with hair spacing; the 2 mm spaces between pubic hairs are equal to the span of the louse's hind legs, with which it grips hairs. Human blood is the only food of these organisms. The louse pierces host skin with its mouth and drinks blood from a capillary. It may remain attached to this site for several hours. The louse dies if it is removed from the host for more than 24 hours.

Eggs (nits) are laid on a hair shaft near the root and remain firmly attached to the hair shaft by a cement-like substance. The eggs hatch after 5 to 10 days, and the organisms then undergo three molts to become adults, which takes an additional 2 to 3 weeks. Mating occurs several hours after lice reach adulthood. Females then lay eggs at the rate of approximately 4 eggs/day for their 3–4 week life span. Ten or fewer adult lice are usually present on a human host at a given time.

Pubic lice infestation occurs in men and women, is found world wide, and occurs in all ethnic groups. It is most frequently found in single persons aged 15–25 years, and is less common in people over age 35.

Pubic lice are transmitted almost exclusively through sexual contact. Pediculosis pubis is more contagious than any other sexually transmitted disease and there is a 95% chance of contracting the infestation from a single sexual encounter. Fomites, such as bedding, may play a minor role in transmission. Animals do not play a role in the transmission of pediculosis pubis.

Evaluation

The clinical manifestations of *Phthirus pubis* infestation are itching and irritation of the pubic area. On occasion patients will have seen lice or nits on their skin or hair. It may take a month to develop symptoms after exposure to an infested partner. This is the time required for growth of the louse population and for development of the host immune response, which is responsible for most of the symptoms. In some cases, when a patient receives many bites over a short period of time, inguinal lympadenopathy, or uncommonly,

---

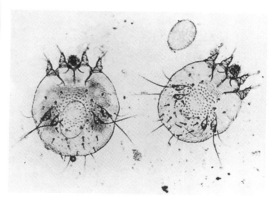

Figure 11.1. *Pediculosis pubis.* Note the claws adapted for grasping hairs. (Reproduced from Rogstad, K.E. et al. *ABC of Sexually Transmitted Infections,* 6th edn. Blackwell Publishing: Oxford, 2011, with permission.)

mild systemic manifestations, such as malaise and low-grade fever, may occur.

Examination reveals the lice or nits in the infested areas. Small erythematous punctate bites are seen near hair follicles. These may resemble folliculitis in some cases. Excoriations and superinfected areas may be seen. Uncommonly, the macula caerulea is seen, a nonblanching painless bluish-gray macule. This is a bite that was followed by a small hemorrhage into the skin.

★ **TIPS & TRICKS**

Patients infested with *Phthirus pubis* may have rust-colored spots on their underclothing the size of a pin head. These represent louse bite sites that have bled, or louse excrement. These may be the first signs that the patient is infested.

There is no laboratory testing for *Phthirus pubis*, and diagnosis relies upon visualizing lice or nits on a patient. A hand lens may be useful in identifying the organisms. Their yellow-gray color may blend in with Caucasian skin and are more easily identified following a blood meal, when they become rust colored. If identified in areas other than the pubic region, they must be distinguished from the human body or head louse by their shape. Microscopy can be used for this purpose. Nits are often easier to see than the organisms themselves and can be distinguished from scales of skin by their firm attachment to the hair shaft. Nits remain adherent to the hair after therapy, and move outward as the hair grows. Such nits do not indicate active infestation; only new nits that are close to the base of the hair shaft are concerning for treatment failure.

Treatment

Centers for Disease Control (CDC)-recommended treatments for *Phthirus pubis* infestation are detailed in Table 11.1.

The affected area should be washed with soap and water and towel-dried prior to the application of medication. Hair should be completely dry prior to the application of lindane shampoo. The medicated lotion, mousse, or shampoo should be applied to the affected areas such that the hair is saturated with the medication, and thoroughly washed off after the appropriate length of time. Following treatment, nits will be killed but will remain attached to the hair shafts and can be removed using a fine-toothed comb.

⚠ **CAUTION!**

Lindane should be avoided in pregnant and breastfeeding women, and also in infants and children, the elderly, persons with a seizure disorder, persons with skin irritation, and persons who weigh less than 110 pounds. It is more easily absorbed or may be more likely to have adverse effects in these populations.

If lice or nits are found on the eyebrows or eyelashes, these medications should not be used. Any visible organisms should be manually removed. Occlusive ophthalmic ointment should be applied to the eyelid margins twice a day for 10 days. Regular petrolatum should not be used, as this can irritate the eyes.

Patients should be re-evaluated one week after treatment if symptoms persist. They should be

Table 11.1. Treatments for Phthirus pubis infestation

Name	Type of patient	Dosage/number of applications	FDA approved	Comments
Permethrin lotion 1%	• Can be used in pregnancy and lactation	• Apply to affected area and wash off after 10 minutes	Y	• Available over-the-counter • Resistance to drug increasing
Pyrethrin and piperonyl butoxide mousse	• Can be used in pregnancy and lactation	• Apply to affected area and wash off after 10 minutes	Y	• Available over-the-counter • Resistance to drug increasing
Lindane shampoo	• Persons who have failed or cannot tolerate other medications • Avoid in infants, children, the elderly, persons with a seizure disorder, pregnant or breast-feeding women, persons with skin irritation, persons who weigh less than 110 pounds	• Apply shampoo directly to dry hair • Work thoroughly into the hair and allow to remain in place for 4 minutes • Then add small amount of water to hair until lather forms • Immediately rinse all lather away	Y	• Prescription only • Not first line therapy due to toxicity
Malathion lotion 0.5%	• Should be used when treatment failure is believed to due to drug resistance	• Apply to affected area and wash off after 8-12 hours	N	• Prescription only • Has bad odor
Ivermectin	• Avoid in pregnant or lactating women	• 200 mcg/kg orally • Repeat dose in 2 weeks • Taken on an empty stomach with water	N	• Oral therapy

retreated if live lice are present or if nits are found at the base of the hair shaft. An alternative regimen should be used for retreatment.

All clothing, towels, and bedding used in the 3 days preceding treatment should be machine washed in hot water (at least 130 °F) and dried in a hot dryer. Items that cannot be washed should be dry cleaned or stored in sealed plastic bags for at least 2 weeks, which kills the organisms.

Partners with whom the patient has had sexual contact within the previous month should also be treated. Patients and partners should avoid sexual contact until both have been re-evaluated and found to be free of infestation. Household contacts do not need to be treated.

Treatment in pregnancy

Pregnant and lactating women should be treated with permethrin (category B) or pyrethrins with piperonyl butoxide (category C). The CDC recommends that lindane and ivermectin should be avoided when possible.

Scabies

Background

Scabies is a dermatosis caused by the human itch mite, *Sarcoptes scabiei* var. *hominis*. The adult female, which is primarily responsible for the rash, is 400 by 300 micrometers in size, translucent, and barely visible to the naked eye (Figure 11.2). It is better visualized with a hand lens.

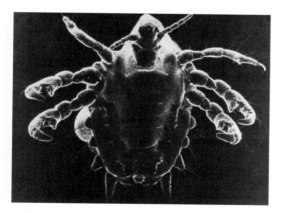

Figure 11.2. *Sarcoptes scabiei.* (Reproduced from Rogstad, K.E. et al. *ABC of Sexually Transmitted Infections,* 6th edn. Blackwell Publishing: Oxford, 2011, with permission.)

The fertilized adult female mite burrows into the outermost layer of the epidermis, the stratum corneum, using its jaws and limbs. It digs through this layer to reach the stratum granulosum, where it lays its eggs. There it feeds on cellular debris and tissue fluid. The mite continues to extend the burrow along the stratum corneum by 0.5 to 5 mm and lays several eggs each day. This process continues for the lifespan of the female, which is 1 to 2 months. After 3 or 4 days, eggs hatch, and the larvae move to the skin surface and create separate burrows called molting pouches. There they undergo several moltings and mature into adult mites within about 10 days. After adult mites copulate within the molting pouches, fertilized females move to the surface of the host skin and begin the process again. The mean number of mites in an infested person is 11, and 50% of patients with scabies are infested with only 1 to 5 mites at a time.

🦠 SCIENCE REVISITED

As the skin of the host constantly turns over, the burrows are pushed nearer to the surface of the skin and eventually slough off. Scratching and bathing accelerate this process, resulting in a relatively low number of mites in the average scabies patient.

Scabies is common throughout the world, and is equally prevalent among men and women. It affects all age groups equally and is seen more often in whites than in blacks.

Sarcoptes scabiei is transmitted by prolonged and steady skin-to-skin contact, so while it can be sexually transmitted, it is often transmitted by other interactions among people. Transmission often occurs within families. In some warm and moist environments, mites can survive away from the host for 2 to 3 days. Therefore, while fomites such as bedding and clothing are not a major source of transmission, the possibility for indirect transmission does exist. *Sarcoptes scabiei* are host-specific, and a strain of the mite infecting one animal cannot efficiently infect another; therefore, most animal-to-human transfers are probably self-limited.

Evaluation

The clinical manifestation of *Sarcoptes scabiei* infestation is a pruritic rash. Symptoms are the result of the host immune response, and require sensitization to mite antigens. Symptoms may therefore take several weeks to appear following an initial infestation. In repeat infestations, symptoms take only 1 to 4 days to develop. The itching is often more intense at night and is worse when the surrounding environment is warm. The mite is most commonly found on the hands and wrists, but is also found on the flexor surfaces of the elbows, the axillae, areolae in women, belt line, buttocks and upper thigh, and the genitalia.

☆ TIPS & TRICKS

Mites are found infesting the wrists and hands in over 80% of cases. The second most common sites are the elbows, feet, and genitalia, each of which is infested about 40% of the time.

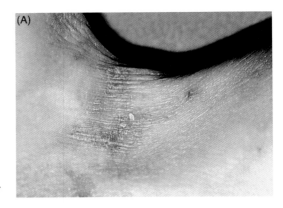

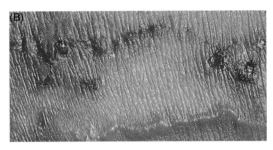

Figure 11.3. (A) and (B) Burrow of the scabies mite in a finger cleft. (Reproduced from Rogstad, K.E. et al. *ABC of Sexually Transmitted Infections,* 6th edn. Blackwell Publishing: Oxford, 2011, with permission.)

Classically, burrows are present, which appear as a gray, thin, serpiginous line, 2–15 mm in length. A small vesicle containing a tiny brown and white mite can be seen at one end of the burrow – see Figures 11.3(A) and (B). More commonly, small erythematous papules with a halo of erythema are seen. Excoriations, nodules, or eczematous lesions can also be seen. Less commonly, urticaria, vasculitis, or superinfected lesions are present. Nodular scabies may be seen rarely. Nodules are firm, reddish-brown, and may persist after treatment. They are filled with an inflammatory infiltrate, and may represent an immunologic reaction to antigens which remain in the skin. Mite parts are often no longer present. A form of scabies called crusted (Norwegian) scabies is seen in immunologically incompetent patients. The thick crusted scales resembling psoriasis are present. Scales often contain large numbers of mites (up to 2 million) and are very contagious.

The diagnosis of scabies should be confirmed via laboratory testing if possible. The sensitivity of these tests often depends upon the skill of the examiner, and ranges from 30 to 90%. Skin scraping, sharp curettage, or shave biopsy of an unexcoriated papule can be performed. The resulting specimen is placed in a drop of mineral oil and examined under the microscope at 50 times magnification. Adult or larval mites, *S. scabiei* eggs, or fecal pellets (scybala) may be seen. Alternately, the ink burrow test can be performed. The papule or burrow is covered with ink from a fountain pen, and the ink is wiped away with alcohol. A positive result is when the ink penetrates the papule and burrow, making a dark wavy line on the skin. Topical tetracycline can be used instead of ink, and a Wood's lamp is used to reveal a yellow-green fluorescent line marking the burrow. The glue stripping test will also be diagnostic in some cases. A drop of methacrylate glue is placed on a glass slide, and the slide is firmly applied to the intact lesion. The glue is allowed to set, then pulled quickly off the lesion. The process is repeated two more times. The slide is then examined under the microscope, and the organisms can be seen. The cellophane tape test employs a similar premise: clear cellophane tape is applied to the skin, and then briskly removed. The tape is placed on a microscope slide. If these methods do not reveal the organism, a punch biopsy can be performed. A 2 mm specimen of an unexcoriated lesion is usually sufficient.

Treatment

CDC-recommended treatments for scabies are detailed in Table 11.2. In most adults and children, the scabicide lotion or cream should be applied to the entire body from the neck down. In infants and debilitated persons, the scabicide should be applied to the entire head and neck as well. Scabicide should be applied to clean skin after bathing, except when treating with lindane.

In most cases, pruritis begins to resolve after 2 days of therapy; however, in some cases, symptoms including rash and pruritis may persist for up to 2 weeks. Symptoms persisting beyond 2 weeks might be due to treatment failure, allergic dermatitis, or an irritant dermatitis from overuse of scabicides. The presence of household mites can also cause symptoms to persist due to cross-reactivity between antigens. Treatment failure can be caused by resistance to scabicides, improper application of scabicides, persistence of mites under fingernails, or reinfection from family members or fomites.

The optimal regimen for treatment of crusted (Norwegian) scabies has not been established. Treatment failure often occurs with a single topical scabicide or oral ivermectin treatment. The CDC suggests dual treatment with a topical scabicide and oral ivermectin on days 1, 2, 8, 9, and 15. Additional treatments with ivermectin on days 22 and 29 may be required. Ivermectin

Table 11.2. Treatments for *Sarcoptes scabiei* infestation

Name	Type of patient	Dosage/number of applications	FDA approved	Comments
Permethrin cream 5%	• Persons at least 2 months of age • Pregnant and lactating women	• 30 g of cream per application • Wash off after 8-14 hours • One application usually curative • 2 or more applications a week apart may be required	Y	• Preferred treatment • Safe and effective
Crotamiton lotion or cream 10%	• Adults • Can be used in children and pregnant and lactating women	• 1 oz of lotion or 30 g of cream per application • Repeat application 24 hours after 1st application • Wash off after additional 48 hours • Second course of therapy often required	Y (adults only)	• Frequent treatment failure reported • Application may give symptomatic relief

(Continued)

Table 11.2. (*Continued*)

Name	Type of patient	Dosage/number of applications	FDA approved	Comments
Lindane lotion 1%	• Avoid in infants, children, the elderly, persons with a seizure disorder, pregnant or breast-feeding women, persons with skin irritation, persons who weigh less than 110 pounds	• 1 oz of lotion or 30 g of cream per application	Y	• Not first line therapy due to toxicity
		• Wash off thoroughly after 8 hours		• Toxicities include CNS toxicity & aplastic anemia
		• Do not apply immediately after bathing		• Low cost
		• One application is usually curative		
		• Second application is recommended if no clinical improvement after 2 weeks		
Ivermectin	• Use in patients who have failed treatment with or who cannot tolerate FDA-approved topical medications	• 200 mcg/kg orally	N	• Oral therapy
	• Safety not established in children weighing less than 15 kg and in pregnant women	• Taken on an empty stomach with water		• More rapid clinical response of pruritis
		• 2 or more doses at least 7 days apart may be required		

should be combined with permethrin cream 5% or benzyl benzoate cream 5%. These topical agents should be applied daily for 7 days and then twice weekly until cured. Lindane should be avoided.

Bedding, clothing, towels and other items used by the infested persons and/or the close contacts should be washed in hot water and dried in a hot dryer, dry-cleaned, or sealed in a plastic bag for at least 72 hours to kill the organisms.

Sexual contacts and household members of the infested person should be treated for scabies. In addition, all other close personal contacts who have had prolonged skin-to-skin contact with the infested person within the last month should be treated. All persons should be treated at the same time to avoid re-infestation. Because scabies may not become symptomatic for several weeks after infestation, it is essential to treat all close contact even if they are asymptomatic.

Treatment in pregnancy

Permethrin is recommended for the treatment of scabies in pregnant or lactating women (category B). The CDC recommends that lindane and ivermectin should be avoided when possible.

Bibliography

http://www.cdc.gov/parasites/Accessed May 3, 2011.

Morse SA, Long J. Infestations. In: *Atlas of Sexually Transmitted Disease and AIDS*, 3rd edn. (Morse SA, et al., eds.). Mosby: Edinburgh, 2003; pp. 349–363.

Orkin M, Maibach HI (eds.). *Cutaneous Infestations and Insect Bites*. Marcel Dekker: New York; 1985.

Sexually Transmitted Diseases Treatment Guidelines. *MMWR* 2010; **59** (RR-12).

Sweet RL, Gibbs RS. (eds.). *Infectious Disease of the Female Genital Tract*, 5th edn. Lippincott Williams & Wilkins: Philadelphia, 2009; pp. 74–76.

Dermatological Conditions and Noninfectious Genital Ulcers

Kathleen McIntyre-Seltman

Department of Obstetrics, Gynecology and Reproductive Sciences, Division of Reproductive Infectious Diseases, Magee-Womens Hospital of the University of Pittsburgh Medical Center, Pittsburgh, PA, USA

Introduction

The vulva is a unique region. It has mucosa, nonhair-bearing, and hair-bearing skin adjacent to each other in a small area. The environment is warm and moist, often with occlusion due to clothing. The sweat glands have chemically different secretions compared with other skin glands. In addition, there may be urine, fecal material, and vaginal secretions which can affect the skin. The vulva is colonized by a wide variety of bacteria, including skin, and vaginal and fecal flora. All these factors conspire to make dermatologic conditions of the vulva look different from elsewhere on the skin, challenging diagnosticians.

Symptoms and evaluation

Approximately 50% of women with vulvar disease are asymptomatic. Symptoms, when they occur, are very nonspecific. Itching, burning, pain, especially with sexual activity, swelling or a lump, or bleeding are the usual symptoms women endorse. Evaluation should consist of a careful inspection and palpation. Although not required, magnification can be extremely helpful in distinguishing areas suspicious for neoplasia and determining biopsy sites. The application of topical agents, such as acetic acid, toluidine blue, or Lugol's iodine solution, has limited use.

Vulvar biopsy is important both to establish an accurate diagnosis and to detect neoplasia. Local anesthesia should be used. Some clinicians prefer topical agents such as EMLA or lidocaine creams; however, these take 30 to 60 minutes to be effective. Lidocaine with or without a vasoconstrictor can be injected using a dental or insulin syringe with the smallest needle available. [Use of a punch biopsy is considered the most useful and accurate means of obtaining tissue for pathological evaluation, with shave biopsies discouraged since evaluation of the underlying dermis is key in making a diagnosis for many vulvar disorders.] Hemostasis can be assured with the application of an astringent solution such as silver nitrate or ferrous subsulfate, or with a fine absorbable suture. Patients should be counseled that astringent solutions may leave dark particles under the skin due to the deposition of metal salts. Ulcers should be biopsied at the edge of the area that is eroded to ensure that some epithelium is included, while nonulcerated lesions should be biopsied from the middle. Small lesions are best removed with an elliptical excision following the skin lines for best cosmetic results (see Box 12.1).

Sexually Transmitted Diseases, First Edition. Edited by Richard H. Beigi.
© 2012 John Wiley & Sons, Ltd. Published 2012 by John Wiley & Sons, Ltd.

Box 12.1. Vulvar biopsy techniques

- Use local anesthesia!
- Avoid shave biopsy.
- Punch biopsy is recommended.
- Obtain hemostasis with silver nitrate, ferrous subsulfate or cautery.
- Suture rarely needed.
- For focal lesions, excisional biopsy may be preferred.

☆ TIPS & TRICKS

Use of a punch biopsy is considered the most useful and accurate means of obtaining tissue for pathological evaluation, with shave biopsies discouraged since evaluation of the underlying dermis is key in making a diagnosis for many vulvar disorders.

Patient concerns

Many women are reluctant to discuss vulvar symptoms with the clinician who cares for them, thus it is important to ask specifically about itching, irritation, burning, soreness, or lesions related to the vulva, as well as asking about pain with sexual activity including touching, oral contact, and/or penetration. It is also important to examine the vulva when performing a routine pelvic examination, since women may have a significant disease but be asymptomatic. Clinicians sometimes think of the vulva as merely a conduit for the speculum, not taking time to separate the labial folds and carefully inspect the introitus.

Women with vulvar symptoms may be afraid as well as embarrassed, and they are usually fearful about the possibility of cancer or a sexually-transmitted origin of the disorder. In addition, vulvar disorders have a significant impact on body image and sexual function. Since many women will not share their concerns, it is important for clinicians to address these issues whether or not the patient mentions them. All women with vulvar disorders should be counseled about the etiology of the condition and the risk (or lack of risk) of sexual transmission. Even if a patient does not endorse sexual activity, a discussion about the effects of sex on the disorder as well as the disorder on sex should be initiated by the clinician. The symptoms associated with vulvar disorders are often exacerbated by sexual activity, including touching and oral sex as well as penetration. Use of topical lidocaine before, during, and after sexual contact can relieve discomfort without a significant effect on a partner. In addition, rinsing with cool water to remove local irritants, and the use of ice packs after sex, may be helpful.

Clinicians caring for women with vulvar disorders need to be alert to the significant psychological distress that often accompanies these conditions. Depression, anxiety, and social isolation can be exacerbated. Sleep disruption due to itching or pain may have functional consequences. Distorted body image may also be an important concern. When dealing with chronic conditions, it is common for women to feel helpless and hopeless. It is important to screen for evidence of disturbed physical and psychologic function during both initial and follow-up visits. Referral to a mental health specialist when indicated is an important part of the care of women with vulvar disorders.

Most women with noninfectious vulvar disorders can obtain moderate relief of symptoms by a simple vulvar care regimen (see Box 12.2). All the topical agents the patient has been using (both prescription and nonprescription) should be discontinued, including steroids, antibiotics, or antifungal agents. Other chemical agents such as soaps, feminine hygiene agents, premedicated adult or baby wipes, and commonly used household chemicals, including vinegar and baking soda, should also be stopped. Most women will find it too inconvenient to soak in a tub, so the vulva and perineum should be cleansed with sitz baths of tepid water, rinsing with a squirt bottle of water or the hose apparatus that comes with the sitz bath. The use of washcloths or sponges should be discouraged, since many women will rub hard enough to injure the skin. Soaking is followed by air drying or drying with a cool hair dryer. Any newly prescribed medications should be applied to clean dry skin. Nonocclusive underwear and clothing are encouraged.

Box 12.2. Vulvar hygiene measures

- Cleanse without soap.
- Soak in sitz bath at least twice daily, using plain *lukewarm* water.
- Dry vulva by gentle patting or with a hair dryer on *cool* setting.
- Apply steroid ointment to clean dry skin.
- Use emollient ointments such as petrolatum or Eucerin® without additives between doses of medication.
- Use lidocaine gel or ointment as needed.
- Use squirt bottle or rinsing instead of toilet tissue after toileting.
- Avoid over the counter medications, creams, cleansing and deodorant products.
- Wash underclothes separately with non scented detergent or soap, dry without fabric softener.
- Avoid tight clothing, occlusive clothing (non-breathable underwear, spandex, panty girdles, tights or pantyhose) and clothing with thick seams in the vulvar region (jeans).
- If possible, avoid underwear and pajama bottoms for sleep.
- Manage incontinence.

Medications for vulvar disorders

Topical steroids are the cornerstone of therapy for many vulvar disorders. Although many clinicians have concerns about the use of very high-potency steroids on the vulva, clinical experience shows that these agents can be used without fear of skin atrophy or striae. For reasons that are unclear, the vulva is quite resistant to the steroid side effects that have been seen on other skin areas. In addition, hyperkeratotic lesions require high-potency steroids to penetrate the thickened epithelium. For these reasons, high-potency agents such as clobetasol are the drug of choice when topical steroids are indicated. Low-potency steroids should be avoided except when used as part of a maintenance regimen after disease control has been achieved. It is critical to counsel patients about the safety of topical steroids, as the package insert and pharmacy instructions usually contain prominent warnings against genital use as well as long-term use. Unless this issue is specifically addressed by the clinician when the medication is prescribed, patients will often be afraid to use it.

☆ TIPS & TRICKS

Women should be directly counseled about the safety of long term use of high-potency topical steroids with certain vulvar dermatologic conditions given contradictory information on the package inserts.

Cream, gel, and lotion vehicles tend to be poorly tolerated on the vulva. They cause irritation and burning with application. Ointment vehicles should almost always be used. It may be necessary to work with a compounding pharmacist when patients have irritant or allergic reactions to preservatives or other agents in a commercially produced medication (see Box 12.3).

Box 12.3. Common vulvar irritants

Physiologic
- Urine.
- Vaginal secretions.
- Stool.
- Perspiration.
- Semen, saliva.

Chemical
- Benzocaine (topical anesthetic, in many OTC medications).
- Chlorhexidine (topical antibacterial, in many OTC medications including K-Y jelly®).
- Preservatives.
- Topical antibiotics (OTC antibacterial creams).
- Vehicle agents in creams and gels.
- Fragrances (in soaps, OTC products).
- Deodorants (for skin use or in sanitary pads).
- Baby or adult moistened wipes.
- Coloring agents in products or clothing.
- Fabric softeners and detergents.
- Depilatory agents.
- Latex.
- Spermicides.

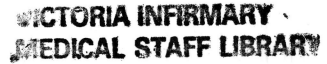

Physical
- Rubbing/scratching.
- Tight clothing/thick seams in clothing.
- Sexual activity.
- Activities with vulvar pressure (bicycle or horse riding).
- Sanitary pads, incontinence pads and panty liners.

For many disorders, topical lidocaine ointment 5% or gel 2% can be a useful adjunct for the control of itching, burning, and pain. Lidocaine can be applied as frequently as needed for symptom relief, and can be especially useful before exercise or sexual activity for women with vulvodynia. Other commonly used topical anesthetics, such as benzocaine, should be avoided because they commonly cause allergic sensitization (see Box 12.4).

Box 12.4. Prescribing medications for vulvar disease

- Prescribe ultrapotent topical steroid ointment.
- Steroid atrophy of vulvar skin is very rare.
- Counsel patient regarding safety of long term use of high-potency steroids.
  - Package insert and pharmacists warn against chronic use.
  - Patients often discontinue use unless these warnings are addressed by the prescribing clinician.
- Begin with BID application to clean dry skin.
- Taper use until least frequent maintenance dose is reached.
- Recommend bland emollient between applications of steroid.
- Other topical/systemic immune modulators may be needed.
- Topical lidocaine gel 2% or ointment 5% can be useful adjunct.

Avoid
- Low-potency steroids.
- Topical antihistamines.
- Topical benzocaine or other OTC analgesics.
- All gels, lotions, and creams.

For women with severe itching, oral antihistamines may be needed, especially before sleep. For those with burning, the administration of amitriptyline, nortriptyline, gabapentin, or pregabalin has been shown to be effective. Patients should be started on low doses before sleep, with gradual dose increases as tolerated.

Specific conditions

Lichen sclerosus

Formerly known as lichen sclerosus et atrophicus, lichen sclerosus is an autoimmune condition preferentially affecting vulvar nonhair-bearing skin. It is occasionally located on the penis, and rarely on other areas of skin. Although the exact etiology of lichen sclerosus is unknown, it has been associated with specific HLA haplotypes and with a family or personal history of other autoimmune conditions. In the past, lichen sclerosus was found to be associated with pernicious anemia; however, at present, it is most commonly associated with Hashimoto's thyroiditis and a positive ANA. Histologically, there is thinning of the epithelium with loss of rete pegs, associated with loss of elastin fibers and a homogeneous band of debris in the upper dermis with varying degrees of chronic inflammation. Itching, burning, and dyspareunia are the most common symptoms reported, but many women report no symptoms, with lichen sclerosus diagnosed on routine physical examination. Typical findings can be noted in Figures 12.1 and 12.2.

The clinical appearance of lichen sclerosus is very characteristic. The affected skin is pale white, with finer than normal skin lines producing a crinkled appearance. There may be hyperkeratosis and erosions, especially if the patient is scratching. Subepithelial bleeding, either appearing as petechiae or larger spider-shaped areas, are common. Generally the skin changes are symmetrical, often extending to the perineum and around the anus in a figure-of-eight distribution. There is often a loss of labia minora and periclitoral phimosis, resulting in the clitoris being completely buried beneath the fused prepuce. The introitus may be significantly restricted from these chronic skin changes.

Management

The most effective treatment for lichen sclerosus is a high–potency topical steroid ointment such as clobetasol applied twice daily to clean dry skin.

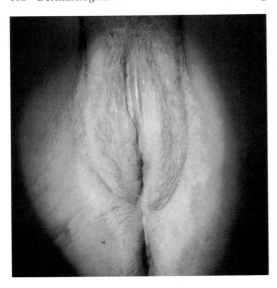

Figure 12.1. Lichen sclerosus.

When symptoms and clinical skin changes have begun to regress, the dose can be gradually tapered to once daily. Since this is an autoimmune condition, prolonged maintenance therapy is usually required once the disease has been initially controlled. Some clinicians switch to low-potency steroid ointments; others continue

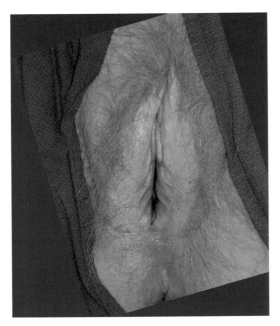

Figure 12.2. Lichen sclerosus.

clobetasol intermittently, with doses as frequently as needed to prevent symptom flares. Many women can be managed with clobetasol two to four times monthly, and emollient use in between. There is an association with squamous cell carcinoma and lichen sclerosus. The magnitude of risk of malignancy is unclear, with estimates of 5% of women with lichen sclerosus ultimately developing cancer in the affected area. Conversely, in at least 50% of women with vulvar carcinoma, lichen sclerosus has been found in adjacent skin on histologic evaluation. It is generally believed, but not proven, that good control of the disorder decreases the risk of malignancy, so women should continue treatment even if they are minimally symptomatic. It is important to continue surveillance by an experienced clinician, with biopsy of any areas that are suspicious for intraepithelial neoplasia or cancer.

High-potency steroid ointment is usually successful at controlling symptoms and clinical appearance of the affected skin. If a woman is poorly responsive to initial therapy, a repeat biopsy should be considered as the diagnosis may be incorrect. When lichen sclerosus is refractory to steroids, a variety of second-line treatments have been used with limited success. These include topical tacrolimus or pimecrolimus, systemic immune suppression with pulse doses of steroids, dapsone, or TNF-modulating drugs such as entarecept or inflixamab. In the past, topical testosterone ointment was the mainstay of therapy; however, this therapy no longer has an accepted role in treatment.

Lichen planus

Lichen planus is a painful autoimmune condition involving the mucosa of the vulva, vagina, and mouth as well as skin, typically on flexor surfaces of the wrists and arms. There is a papular form and an erosive form, the latter of which is more common on the vulva. The cause is unknown. On mucosal surfaces, the lesions are usually erosive, with loss of superficial epithelium. They are very tender to touch, and bleed readily with contact. On the skin, the lesions typically appear as small pale purple polygonal papules, although there may also be erosive and crusting lesions. As the erosions heal, there are often weblike lacy white strands of epithelium covering the eroded areas, known as Wickham's striae. There is often contracture of affected tissue and coaptation of adjacent eroded surfaces. The vagina may become completely obliterated, and the labia may be so tightly adherent that urination becomes difficult.

The diagnosis of lichen planus can often based on the typical appearance and distribution of the lesions. It is important to search for vaginal lesions, which appear as beefy red eroded areas associated with a blood-tinged purulent appearing discharge. Oral lesions are usually located on the gums, soft palate, or inner cheek. Biopsy findings are nonspecific and may not be diagnostic, but are still important to rule out other conditions such as bullous diseases, VIN, or Paget's disease.

Lichen planus is best managed with a topical high-potency steroid ointment such as clobetasol. Creams should be avoided as they can cause severe burning on the eroded lesions. Most women need at least daily or twice daily steroid ointment to obtain control of the erosions. If topical steroids cause too much pain on application, a short course of high-dose systemic prednisone may be required before topical agents can be reintroduced. Vaginal lesions can be treated with hydrocortisone suppositories (marketed for rectal use) or with clobetasol inserted into the vagina with an applicator such as that used for antifungal or hormone preparations. Since this is an autoimmune disorder, treatment is continued indefinitely. Lichen planus can be very difficult to control, and systemic therapy may be indicated, especially in the patient with extensive oral or skin involvement. High-dose systemic steroids, immune modulators such as cyclosporine or tacrolimus, TNF inhibitors, and thalidomide are often used to control systemic disease. In the woman with refractory lichen planus, comanagement with a dermatologist can be very helpful. In extreme cases, surgery may be needed as an adjunct if there is labial agglutination, urethral obstruction, or vaginal agglutination and obliteration. Usually there are no recognizable tissue planes, so care must be taken not to injure underlying bowel or bladder as the coapted tissues are separated. Given the rarity of these procedures and the technical challenges, it is suggested that only experienced gynecologic surgeons should undertake these procedures.

Squamous cell hyperplasia

Formerly known as hyperplastic dystrophy, squamous cell hyperplasia is now understood to be a form of lichen simplex chronicus. Unlike the autoimmune disorders above, this condition is a response to chronic irritation of the skin, resulting in a thickening of the epidermis, often with abnormal keratinization, and an inflammatory infiltrate in the dermis. Women usually present with severe itching, frequently leading to the disruption of sleep and limitation of usual activities. The lesions can be recognized by their thickened, leathery appearance, with coarsening of the normal skin lines. They may appear white or gray if keratinized, red, or darkly pigmented. Erosions and excoriations from scratching are often seen. Squamous cell hyperplasia lesions generally have an asymmetrical distribution, and can be located anywhere on the skin of the groin, vulva, perineum, or perianal areas (Figures 12.3 and 12.4). Biopsy is indicated because these lesions cannot be distinguished grossly from VIN or malignancy.

The etiology of this disorder is chronic irritation. The skin changes can be initiated by mechanical irritation – for example, tight-fitting clothing, infection, or chemical irritants from perfumes, soaps, laundry products, topical creams, incontinence etc. (see Box 12.2). Continued scratching and continued application of

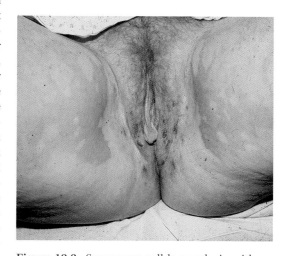

Figure 12.3. Squamous cell hyperplasia with excoriations and post inflammatory depigmentation.

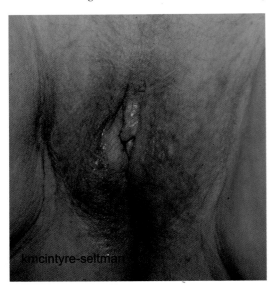

Figure 12.4. Squamous cell hyperplasia with mild hyperkeratosis.

topical agents can perpetuate the inflammatory reaction, until the skin is very abnormal and often thickly keratinized. The inciting factors do not need to continue once the inflammatory process is established, so it is often not possible to identify the offending agents.

Management of squamous cell hyperplasia is aimed at decreasing local irritation and preventing scratching. Vulvar hygiene measures (see Box 12.2) are very helpful in relieving itching and allowing the skin to heal. The patient should be counseled to discontinue the use of all local medications, chemicals, soaps, laundry additives, etc., because many women with squamous cell hyperplasia have become sensitized to topical preservatives, fragrances, and medications. Using a squirt bottle instead of a toilet tissue when possible can be helpful. If the skin is highly keratinized, high-potency topical steroids such as clobetasol are indicated; if the skin is less thickened, then intermediate-potency steroids may be adequate. Ointments are better tolerated than creams, ass creams have more preservatives that may contribute to local irritation. Most of the time, these lesions will regress after several weeks of local care and steroid ointment. The steroids can be tapered rapidly and discontinued, and replaced by emollient ointments such as petro-

latum or Eucerin®. Unlike the autoimmune vulvar disorders, squamous cell hyperplasia usually does not require maintenance steroid therapy, although intermittent topical steroids may be needed for recurrences.

Contact irritation and allergy

Because the vulva remains moist and functionally occluded by clothing and body habitus, contact sensitization is common. This can take the form of true contact allergy, in which a previously sensitized person develops a dermatitis resembling poison ivy 24 to 48 hours after exposure to the allergen. More common is contact irritation without allergy, which usually occurs soon after exposure. Irritant reactions vary tremendously in appearance, ranging from subtle erythema to blistering. The skin is often lichenified, but may be normal in texture with minimal color change. The lesions are usually ill defined with indistinct borders, and may be anywhere on the vulva. It is usually very difficult to identify the offending agent(s), especially after the irritation has become chronic. Biopsy findings are nonspecific, with varying epithelial thickening and blunting of rete pegs, spongiosis, and chronic inflammation.

The list of agents that can cause contact irritant or allergy is extensive. Medications including topical steroids, local anesthetics (especially benzocaine), and chemicals found in feminine hygiene products and depilatories are common irritants. Metals, especially nickel, can cause allergy on the vulva just as it can anywhere else. Consider nickel allergy if there is ongoing irritation around vulvar piercings or "jewelry." Preservatives and vehicle chemicals in creams, lotions, soaps and other agents can be both irritants and allergens. Laundry products, particularly liquid or dryer sheet fabric softeners, are designed to stay in fabrics and can be irritating.

Management is aimed at decreasing all local irritation. If the specific irritant or allergen can be identified, it is fairly straightforward to avoid contact with it. Most of the time, however, it is impossible to identify the inciting agents. Treatment should begin with discontinuation of all topical medications, creams, soaps, laundry additives, and other products. The patient should soak in tepid water at least twice daily and protect dry skin with Eucerin® or petrolatum. If there is severe irritation or blistering, an intermediate or high-potency steroid ointment can be used twice daily. A short course of high-dose systemic steroids may be needed, especially if topical steroids are too painful to use or are not entirely successful. All creams, lotions, and over-the-counter steroids should be avoided. If a contact reaction to steroids is suspected, it may be necessary to have a pharmacist compound a steroid ointment in a vehicle without preservatives or irritants. It is challenging for the patient to avoid contact with all potential irritants, but every effort should be made to do so. Measures that can be helpful include (a) washing with just water or a mild, nonfragranced superfatted soap such as Basis®, (b) washing underwear separately with a mild soap and no fabric softeners, and (c) the avoidance of pads and panty liners. Because incontinence is often a contributing factor to local irritation either because of urine or diaper products, efforts to manage urine loss with medication, pelvic floor rehabilitation, or surgery are valuable. If a true contact allergy is suspected, patch testing by an allergist or dermatologist may be indicated.

Hidradenitis suppurativa

Hidradenitis suppurativa is an inflammatory disorder characterized by painful deep subcutaneous nodules which rupture, creating deep interconnected sinuses and healing with significant scar. This disorder involves the axilla and vulva, and less commonly the inframammary folds. This disorder is rare before puberty and generally presents in the 20s. While the drainage from the nodules appears purulent, it seldom grows any organisms on culture. The lesions may cause more pain than would be expected given their appearance. The etiology of hidradenitis suppurativa is unknown; it was thought to be related to apocrine sweat glands but is now thought to be a response to an obstruction of the pilosebaceous unit. There is a genetic component, with about one-third of affected patients having at least one other family member affected. Hidradenitis suppurativa can be diagnosed by the typical appearance and distribution of lesions coupled with a chronic, relapsing course and scarring.

Management

Medical management of hidradenitis suppurativa has limited success. The vulva should be cleansed with an antibacterial soap at least twice daily. Topical antibiotics, particularly clindamycin, have been evaluated with equivocal results. Chronic oral antibiotics such as fluroquinolones, tetracyclines, ampicillin-clavulinic acid, or clindamycin are generally prescribed, although the efficacy of antibiotic therapy has not been proven. Women of reproductive age should be counseled about pregnancy prevention when on tetracyclines and fluoquinolones. Hormonal strategies to decrease androgens have been found to decrease the frequency and severity of the lesions. Women of child-bearing age can be managed with nonandrogenic oral contraceptives (or ring or patch equivalents) or with GnRH agonists for severe disease. In the past, retinoic acid derivatives have been used with modest success; however, these are not currently available. Recently, TNF inhibitors have been used for severe disease with reports of efficacy. Because this is a chronic condition, ongoing therapy is generally needed. If antibiotics are part of the regimen, they may need to be changed periodically.

Surgical approaches are the mainstay of management for moderate to severely advanced cases. Isolated lesions can be unroofed under local anesthesia in the office. More often, larger areas require extensive resection of the nodules and sinus tracts in the operating room with regional or general anesthesia. All affected tissue should be excised, including the inflamed subcutaneous tissues and the overlying skin. It is important to leave no sinus tracts. This often results in very extensive wounds, which may require tissue flaps if the wound cannot be closed. Extensively debrided areas may be left open or managed with a wound vacuum device. Recurrences are common, especially during the reproductive years. Close follow-up to detect and treat small areas of disease may decrease the need for repeated extensive resections. Again, surgeons with experience in such cases are advised.

Other dermatologic disorders

Common dermatologic conditions such as eczema and psoriasis may look very different on the vulva compared with other body regions. In general, scaling is rare on the vulva because of the chronic moisture. Lesions that tend to have scale

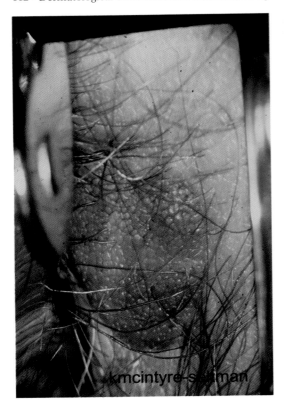

Figure 12.5. Seborrheic keratosis.

elsewhere on the body often appear on the vulva as shiny mildly edematous red patches. It is important to evaluate all the patient's skin, especially flexor surfaces (eczema) and extensor surfaces over joints (psoriasis), as well as the scalp (seborrheic dermatitis). The differential diagnosis is wide, and includes the range of dermatologic conditions, infection with *Candida* or dermatophytes, VIN, and the autoimmune diseases. One lesion occasionally noted on the vulvar area is seborrheic keratosis (Figure 12.5). Careful history, physical examination, cultures for infections, and biopsy when indicated, can all be helpful in making a diagnosis. Consultation and comanagement with a dermatologist is often beneficial for women with dermatoses affecting the vulva.

Psoriasis

Psoriatic lesions on the vulva rarely show the thick silver scale characteristic of lesions found elsewhere on the body. The vulvar lesions tend to be deep red and sharply demarcated with serpiginous borders. Psoriasis may be confused with cutaneous candidiasis or Paget's disease. It is unusual for a woman to have psoriasis only on the vulva, so a general physical examination is important in making the diagnosis. Management is the same as psoriasis elsewhere, with systemic therapy indicated for widespread disease. Topical steroids can be used intermittently but ongoing chronic use should be avoided. Locally, tar derivatives and UV light therapy can be use, but systemic treatment with methotrexate or TNF inhibitors is frequently needed.

Eczema and seborrheic dermatitis

These conditions are less common on the vulva than elsewhere on the body. The lesions are ill defined, usually thickened and red or yellowish. The typical thin scale of eczema and thicker yellow greasy scale of seborrheic dermatitis are seldom fully developed on the vulva. Diagnosis is not difficult when the patient has typical lesions elsewhere on her body or scalp, but may require biopsy if systemic lesions are not evident. Management consists of local care, topical steroids, and antiseborrheic lotions as needed.

Bullous diseases

Any of the bullous diseases, such as pemphigus, pemphigoid, and their variants, can involve the vulva, but it is uncommon that the vulva is the only site of the disease. These are thought to be autoimmune conditions, with antibodies against various components of the squamous epithelium and basement membrane of the epidermis. The resulting immune interaction results in separation of the epidermis and collection of serous fluid between the layers. The bullous disorders can involve both skin and mucous membranes, and may involve the vagina.

Bullous pemphigoid is the most common of these disorders. It usually has its onset in the elderly, and up to 10% of affected women have vulvar involvement. The lesions begin as areas of erythema and edema, progressing to large tense bullae, which rupture and leave painful erosions. Pemphigus has a similar appearance but the bullae are more flaccid, and when tension is applied to adjacent skin, the epidermis slips along the dermis, the Nikolsky sign. Cicatricial pemphigoid is a variant in which the blisters heal with contracting scar. This disorder frequently involves the mouth and eyes. Vulvar and vaginal stenosis may be severe, limiting sexual activity. Hailey–Hailey disease (benign familial pemphigus) is an autosomal dominant disorder which is associated with ulceration of the vulva and vagina, axillae, and inframammary folds. Blistering is seldom seen, and women generally present in their teens and twenties with painful ulceration and scarring.

Bullous diseases are best managed in concert with a dermatologist, since most women will have systemic disease. High-potency topical steroid ointments are used locally on the lesions, and frequently systemic immune suppressant regimens are also needed. Vulvar hygiene, very gentle cleansing, and ice packs are useful adjuncts to manage the erosions. Dilator therapy as well as surgery may be needed in women with cicatricial pemphigoid.

Vulvar ulcers

Ulceration of the vulva can be a difficult problem to diagnose and manage. Ulcers are defined as loss of tissue extending into the epidermis, where erosions involve only the epithelium. Ulcers may be due to infection, autoimmune disorders, contact allergy, malignancy, bullous diseases, underlying disorders such as Crohn's disease, fistulae, trauma, and other conditions. Usually women with vulvar ulcers will present acutely with pain, swelling, and drainage. A more indolent course can be seen with cancer and syphilis. The evaluation of a woman with vulvar ulceration starts with a complete history and physical examination, looking for signs and symptoms of systemic illness, underlying medical conditions, and dermatologic lesions elsewhere on the skin or other mucus membranes. The mouth and perianal areas should be examined carefully. Specimens for culture or antigen identification of infections associated with ulcers should be obtained. Biopsy of ulcers should include the edge of the denuded area with some surrounding skin if possible. In addition to routine histology, immune staining is often needed to make a diagnosis. It is important to communicate with the laboratory, because some immunologic testing requires special tissue handling, such that the biopsy specimen needs to be divided by the clinician, with part placed in formalin or other preservative and part handled differently. Sometimes these lesions are so tender that examination and biopsy under sedation may be required. Serology for specific disorders and infectious agents is often indicated. Symptomatic management with sitz baths, ice packs, and lidocaine gel or ointment can be initiated even if the diagnosis is uncertain.

Sexually transmitted causes of vulvar ulcers are covered in other chapter in this text. The more common noninfectious vulvar ulcers are considered here.

Lipschutz ulcers

These are large painful ulcers involving the labia minora, particularly in children and adolescents. They are thought to be viral in origin, and have been associated with Ebstein–Barr virus infection as well as with a variety of other viruses. It is not clear whether these lesions represent direct mucosal infection or a component of a systemic inflammatory response. The ulcers typically resolve spontaneously over days to weeks. Management is aimed at symptom control, with topical lidocaine gel or ointment, ice packs, and pain medication. Neither topical nor systemic steroids have been shown to be useful.

Aphthous ulcers

While less common on the vulva than the oral mucosa, aphthous ulcers may be recurrent and quite painful. Most commonly, these lesions resemble herpes infections, presenting as multiple blisters which open into punched-out appearing painful ulcers with intensely red bases (Figure 12.6). Sometimes, however, they can form large ulcers involving the entire labia. Because aphthous ulcers can be recurrent and tend to favor the same location, it is important to do testing to rule out herpes. Although the etiology of aphthous ulcers is considered by some to be viral, no causative organisms have been identified or characterized. These lesions will resolve spontaneously, usually within days. Topical high-potency steroids are often used, but it is unclear whether they hasten healing. Symptom-

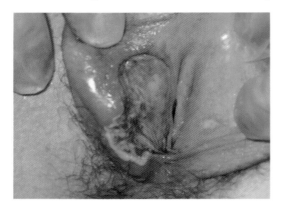

Figure 12.6. Aphthous ulcer in adolescent.

atic management is similar to that for Lipschutz ulcers, described above.

Behçet's disease

This autoimmue disorder is characterized by painful and destructive ulcers of the vulva and oral mucosa, along with iritis/uveitis. The ulcers cause scarring and tissue destruction, sometimes leaving fenestrations in the labia minora. Systemic manifestations are common, including arthritis, cerebritis which may present with neurologic deficits or psychiatric symptoms, and intestinal dysfunction. Behçet's eye disease may cause blindness. Populations most commonly affected are those of middle eastern and eastern Mediterranian origin, with Turkey being the country with the highest prevalence. Acute episodes of ulceration generally respond within a few days to a pulse of high-dose prednisone. Chronic treatment includes high-potency topical steroids if tolerated by the patient, along with systemic immune suppression with steroids, methotrexate, tacrolimus, and TNF antagonists. As Behçet's disease is a multiorgan disorder, coordination with other specialists is important in its management.

Crohn's disease

This disease may involve the vulva as well as the perianal area. Typically the lesions are longitudinal painful deep ulcers, described as "knifelike," in the interlabial sulci. These lesions are distinct from fistulous tracts, which may also involve the vulva, most commonly the labia majora. Perianal fissures or fistulae are often present when there is labial disease. Vulvar manifestations of Crohn's disease may be the presenting symptoms of the disorder, antedating inflammatory bowel symptoms by months to years. Biopsy will show noncaseating granulomata and inflammation. Vulvar Crohn's disease responds poorly to topical therapy and is best treated with systemic immune suppression. High-dose prednisone will usually control the lesions rapidly, with transition to chronic immune modulation with other agents for long-term management. Surgical resection may be needed if fistulae are present. Even if the patient has no bowel symptoms at the time vulvar Crohn's disease is diagnosed, consultation with a gastroenterologist is indicated.

Pyoderma granulosum

The lesions are rapidly enlarging, deep, painful ulcers associated with a dark red edematous border. Usually this disorder is associated with systemic disease, particularly inflammatory bowel disease, lymphoma, and leukemia, but it may appear on the vulva in the absence of other conditions. The lesions of pyoderma granulosum are often mistaken for infection or malignancy, and biopsy is usually needed to confirm the diagnosis. The lesions can regress with systemic steroid management, but often the associated systemic disorder must be controlled before the vulvar lesions remit.

Other

Vulvar ulceration can be present in a variety of other systemic disorders. It is uncommon for the vulvar lesions to be the presenting features of these diseases; usually, vulvar ulceration is associated with other manifestations of active systemic disease. Autoimmune conditions such as lupus erythematosis and scleroderma, and neoplasms such as lymphoma or leukemia occasionally produce deep vulvar ulcers. Graft versus host disease may cause extensive vulvar and vaginal erosions and ulceration, with obliteration of normal tissue during healing. Ulcers associated with systemic disease will resolve as the systemic disease is controlled. Symptomatic management can be a significant clinical challenge, as these lesions can be very painful and difficult to control. Patients may require opoids and other pain medication adjuncts.

Summary

The vulva is a unique environment where hair-bearing skin, glabrous (nonhair-bearing) skin, and mucosa come together. Flora normally found in the skin, vagina, and rectum are all present, and the area is moist and functionally occluded. These factors conspire to make diagnosis and management of vulvar disorders challenging. A few overriding principles apply:

- Biopsy liberally.
- Decrease local irritation.
- Use high-potency steroid ointments when steroids are indicated.
- Attend to psychological and sexual function concerns.
- Work with dermatologists and other specialists as needed.

Bibliography

ACOG. Practice Bulletin No. 93: Diagnosis and management of vulvar skin disorders. *Obstet Gynecol* 2008; **111**: 1243.

Farage MD. Vulvar susceptibility to contact irritants and allergens: a review. *Arch Gynecol Obstet* 2005; **210**: 167.

Journal. *Dermatologic Clinics* 2010; **28** (4). [Entire October 2010 issue is devoted to vulvar disease. Each chapter is an excellent review of a specific disorder by recognized experts.]

Lewis FM. An overview of vulvar ulceration. *Clin Obstet/Gynecol* 2005; **48**: 824.

Margesson LJ. Vulvar disease pearls. *Dermatol Clin* 2006; **24**: 145.

Pels R, et al. Clobetasol propionate – where, when, why? *Drugs Today* 2008; **44**: 547.

Wilkinson EJ, Stone IK. *Atlas of Vulvar Disease*, 2nd edn., 2008. [Outstanding photographs and succinct clinical summaries.]

Vulvodynia

Glenn Updike

Department of Obstetrics, Gynecology and Reproductive Sciences,
Division of Reproductive Infectious Diseases, Magee-Womens Hospital of the
University of Pittsburgh Medical Center, Pittsburgh, PA, USA

Introduction

Providers of women's healthcare will frequently encounter patients with chronic vulvovaginal symptoms with no obvious underlying etiology or physical examination findings. Although these patients describe troublesome and debilitating symptoms such as vulvar burning, stinging, irritation, or rawness, subsequent testing for infection or dermatoses is negative or nonspecific. These cases of otherwise unexplained chronic vulvar discomfort represent a syndrome called "vulvodynia". Vulvodynia is defined by the International Society for the Study of Vulvovaginal Disease (ISSVD) as "vulvar discomfort, most often described as burning pain, occurring in the absence of relevant visible findings or a specific, clinically identifiable, neurologic disorder." An understanding of vulvodynia is important to those involved in the care of women as this syndrome has a profound impact on sexuality, relationships, and quality of life. This chapter outlines what is currently understood about vulvodynia and highlights diagnostic and management considerations for affected patients.

Background and nomenclature

Although vulvodynia has only recently become an area of active clinical and research interest, descriptions of the syndrome can be found in textbooks dating to the eighteen hundreds. These early textbooks discussed a condition of hyperesthesia of the vulva, and the following century saw many terms used to describe the condition. Depending on the time period, vulvodynia was variably known by such terms as dysesthetic vulvodynia, vulvar dysesthesia, and commonly as vulvar vestibulitis. As understanding of the syndrome has progressed, and the nomenclature for vulvodynia has been accordingly refined.

> ### SCIENCE REVISITED
>
> **Pain terminology**
> Allodynia: Pain due to a stimulus that does not normally provoke pain
> Dysesthesia: An unpleasant abnormal sensation, whether spontaneous or evoked
> Hyperalgesia: An increased pain from a stimulus that normally causes pain
> Hyperesthesia: Increased sensitivity to stimulation, excluding the special senses

The most recent terminology, established by the 2003 World Congress of the ISSVD, divides vulvodynia into a generalized and localized variant, with each variant being subcategorized as

Sexually Transmitted Diseases, First Edition. Edited by Richard H. Beigi.
© 2012 John Wiley & Sons, Ltd. Published 2012 by John Wiley & Sons, Ltd.

Table 13.1. 2003 ISSVD Classification and Terminology of Vulvodynia

Vulvar pain related to a specific disorder
• Infectious
• Inflammatory
• Neoplastic
• Neurologic
Vulvodynia
Generalized
• Provoked (sexual, nonsexual, and both)
• Unprovoked
• Mixed (provoked and unprovoked)
Localized
• Provoked (sexual, nonsexual, and both)
• Unprovoked
• Mixed (provoked and unprovoked)

Source: Moyal-Barracco M, Lynch PJ. 2003 ISSVD terminology and classification of vulvodynia: a historical perspective. *J Repro Med* 2004; **49**(10): 772–777.

either provoked or unprovoked (Table 13.1). What was previously known as "vulvar vestibulitis" is now called localized, provoked vulvodynia. Although clinicians still frequently use the term vulvar vestibulitis, it should be abandoned as it incorrectly implies an infectious or inflammatory etiology for the syndrome.

Incidence

It is difficult to know the true incidence of vulvodynia as many women with vulvar pain are either misdiagnosed or never seek care for their symptoms. A population-based assessment of women in the greater Boston area estimated the prevalence of unexplained chronic vulvar pain and found that 16% of respondents reported a history suggestive of vulvodynia, and about 7% of respondents were experiencing symptoms at the time of the survey. Of note, 40% of women that reported chronic vulvar pain responded that they had never sought care for their symptoms. Of those that did seek care, 60% responded that they saw three or more doctors in an effort to relieve their symptoms. Other investigators have noted a similar prevalence of vulvodynia even when the diagnosis is confirmed by physical examination.

> ☆ **TIPS & TRICKS 1**
>
> ***Physical examination***
> Assess the entire vulva by lightly touching the area with a cotton-tip applicator. Ask the patient to tell you where she is having pain, and whether the pain is spontaneous or worsened with touch. Record the examination findings on a diagram of the vulva in the patient's medical record.

Etiology

Despite decades of clinical research, the cause of vulvodynia remains unknown. Although no single factor has been isolated as an etiology, psychological, dietary, infectious, inflammatory, and neuropathic causes have all been postulated.

Psychological factors

Women with vulvodynia experience pain that limits their ability to have intercourse. Understandably, the inability to have pleasurable sex without pain could be a source of stress in a relationship, especially if the partner is not sensitive to the impact of vulvodynia on sexuality. While there is surely physiologic evidence that women with vulvodynia have elevated levels of stress and diminished quality of life, there does exist a "chicken or the egg" argument. That is, did life stressors such as depression, sexual abuse, or physical abuse cause a women to develop chronic vulvar pain, or does the existence of vulvar pain in itself result in psychological distress?

The risk of major depressive disorder (MDD) is higher in women with vulvodynia, with a lifetime prevalence rate of about 45%. Many women report that their first episode of depression preceded the onset of vulvodynia. Psychological distress has been noted in women seeking care in a referral center for vulvar disorders, with vulvodynia patients scoring significantly higher on psychometric testing than women with other vulvar pathology. However, not all studies have demonstrated an increased prevalence of psychological distress among women with vulvodynia. One investigation compared women with a confirmed diagnosis of vulvodynia with women seen in a chronic pelvic pain clinic, as well as asymptomatic women in a general gynecology clinic. Although depression was fairly common in all three groups, the patients with vulvodynia did not differ from the control group in past depression history or in other measures of psychological distress, with both groups having less psychological distress than the chronic pelvic pain group. Another investigation demonstrated that women with localized, provoked vulvodynia generally appear to be psychologically healthy. While the evidence is conflicting, therapies that exclusively target psychological symptoms in women with vulvodynia are probably misguided and insufficient.

As with markers of psychological distress, there is conflicting evidence as to the prevalence of abuse in women with vulvodynia. Population-based evaluations of abuse in women with vulvodynia have shown that adult-onset vulvodynia is strongly associated with both childhood physical and sexual abuse. However, other clinic-based investigations have not consistently confirmed this association of abuse and vulvodynia. These findings highlight that while most women presenting for care for vulvar pain will not have a history of physical or sexual abuse, it is important to screen for abuse in patients with vulvodynia and to offer appropriate counseling services to those that are screen positive.

Dietary factors

There is no clear link between dietary factors and subsequent development of vulvodynia. Based on a single case report describing improvement in vulvodynia symptoms after following a low oxalate diet, many clinicians continue to advise their patient to follow this restrictive diet. Subsequent investigations found, however, that when women with vulvodynia were compared with asymptomatic controls, there was no difference in the urinary excretion of oxalates. Further, when women with vulvodynia with higher oxalate excretion are placed on a low oxalate diet, their symptoms do not reliably improve. Hence, clinicians should carefully evaluate whether initiating a restrictive diet on their patients with vulvodynia is justified, given the lack of evidence for a correlation between oxalates and vulvodynia.

Infection

To date, there is no clear evidence that vulvodynia is an infectious process. Women with a self-reported history of infection and a clinical diagnosis of vulvodynia have more self-reported yeast and urinary tract infections when compared with controls. While existing data does not support an infectious etiology of vulvodynia, it is possible that an infection could set off a cascade of events that ultimately results in vulvodynia and continued vulvar pain even upon resolution of the infection.

Inflammation

Inflammation may contribute to the development of vulvodynia symptoms, but as with other proposed etiologies, the existing evidence is inconclusive. Compared with women not experiencing vulvar pain, biopsies of vulvar tissue in women with vulvodynia show more inflammatory cells (generally a lymphocytic infiltrate) and mast cells. A number of studies have assessed inflammatory mediators in women with vulvodynia. Interestingly some of these studies have shown no increase in mediators such as TNF-α and IL-1, but other investigations have shown slightly elevated levels of the same mediators. While it is difficult to draw a definitive conclusion about the role of inflammation in vulvodynia, mounting evidence suggests that inflammation is of marginal importance, at best, in causing this syndrome. By extension, anti-inflammatory treatments such as steroids are likely to be ineffective in managing symptoms.

Neuropathy

Rather than existing as pathology localized to the vulva, vulvodynia may in fact be a centrally mediated pain phenomenon. Women suffering from vulvodynia have been found to have heightened sensitivity elsewhere on the body, suggesting some systemic disturbance in pain sensation. Additionally, women with vulvodynia have an increased number of nerve endings in the vulvar region compared to controls, further implicating abnormal innervation as an etiologic factor.

Diagnosis

Patients with chronic vulvar pain complaints frequently become frustrated with misdiagnoses and seek care with multiple providers before a correct diagnosis is made. As such, it is vitally important to perform a thorough history, a comprehensive physical examination, and appropriate laboratory evaluation to make an appropriate diagnosis and guide the management plan.

In addition to a comprehensive general medical, gynecologic, and sexual history, it is necessary to obtain the details of the patient's vulvar pain history. The provider must understand the timing of onset of the patient's vulvar pain to distinguish primary vulvodynia (pain with first attempted intercourse or tampon insertion) from secondary vulvodynia that developed after some pain-free interval. Primary vulvodynia likely has a less favorable prognosis than secondary vulvodynia. It is also important to note how long the patient's symptoms have been present. The patient should be questioned as to the nature of her pain; specifically, the patient should be asked to characterize the pain with such terms as "burning," "stabbing," "sharp," or "dull." Of note, various validated measures of the nature and severity of pain have been established, and these questionnaires can be used to follow the course of therapy. The patient should be further questioned as to the variability in intensity of vulvar symptoms and should be asked to specify if the pain is constant or intermittent. Further, it is extremely important to ascertain if the vulvar symptoms are present only with contact (be it with intercourse or tampon insertion) and the degee to which the patient is having symptoms even without contact. Pain that is present only with contact is then classified as *provoked* vulvodynia, while pain occurring in the absence of contact is described as *unprovoked* vulvodynia.

While obtaining the history from women with vulvodynia, the provider must also question the general lifestyle practices of the patient. The use of over-the-counter products should be assessed, including the use of vaginal yeast preparations and feminine hygiene products. The use of benzocaine-containing products has been linked to vulvar pathology and should be noted. It should also be determined if the patient douches, as this may be disruptive to the normal vaginal floura. Assessment of the patient's vulvar hygiene practices should also include questions about the soaps the patient uses, as certain products

– especially those that are heavily scented – could potentially cause vulvar irritation. For similar reasons, the patient should be questioned about the use of laundry detergents and fabric softeners.

☆ TIPS & TRICKS 2

Vulvar care measures

- Wearing cotton underwear, or at least underwear with a cotton crotch
- Do not wear underwear at night
- Avoid scented or fragranced soaps, shampoos, and detergents
- Avoid fabric softeners
- Do not douche
- Use only unscented pads
- Consider using ice packs on the vulva for comfort, but not directly on the skin. Rather, wrap the ice pack in a towel or other fabric before applying and do not leave it on for more than 20 minutes.

Beyond the general physical and usual gynecologic examinations, an extended vulvar assessment should be performed. There should be a careful visual inspection of the vulva from the mons to the perianal region, and laterally from the left to right genitocrural folds. Particular attention should be given to the skin and architecture of the labia majora and the labia minora, with care to inspect the intralabial sulci as well. The clitoris and clitoral hood should also be assessed for any changes in skin color or texture. Vulvodynia is a diagnosis of exclusion, so dermatologic findings would suggest a different etiology for the patient's vulvar pain.

The vulvar vestibule (defined as the area proximal to the labia minora but distal to the hymeneal ring) represents the most common region of symptoms for localized vulvodynia, and, as such, should be carefully assessed. Areas of erythema in the vestibule may be found in patients with vulvodynia. A cotton-tip applicator should be used to assess the entire vulva and vestibule. The patient should be asked to report where on the vulva she experiences pain with a light touch of this cotton-tip applicator, and the findings should be documented in the patient's record. Digital examination of the vagina should include particular attention to the muscles surrounding the vagina. Muscle spasm and tenderness are often noted and this finding may help to guide the management plan.

The importance of laboratory assessment in this setting is primarily in ruling out other treatable causes of chronic vulvar pain that would preclude a diagnosis of vulvodynia. Microscopy with saline wet mount and potassium hydroxide is important to assess for the presence of bacterial vaginosis, yeast vaginitis, atrophic vaginitis, and desquamative inflammatory vaginitis. While a general vaginal culture appears to have little value, a vaginal culture to assess for yeast can compensate for the fairly low sensitivity of microscopy alone in detecting yeast, and can also allow for speciation. Additionally, a Gram stain can be performed to assess for bacterial vaginosis. Many providers will also rule out cervical sexually-transmitted pathogens at the initial visit for completeness, although these conditions typically are not causes of vulvar pain syndromes.

Treatment

As a single cause of vulvodynia remains unknown, planning a therapeutic regimen for patients can be challenging. There are few randomized-controlled trials available to guide management decisions, and those that do exist often fail to show a treatment effect that is greater than placebo. Providers, therefore, rely on previous experience, case series, and expert opinion in formulating management plans. Experts in the field of vulvovaginal disorders have developed treatment algorithms to aid clinicians in deciding how to treat their patients (Figure 13.1).

Before starting any treatment regimen, it is important to inform patients that a cure for vulvodynia is sometimes not possible. Rather, it is more likely that the patient and her care team will find some treatment that decreases symptoms to a point that is more tolerable and results in an overall improved quality of life. Additionally, it is important to remind patients of the side effects related to her particular treatment regimen. Setting realistic therapeutic goals with an understanding of likely side effects will enhance the patient's treatment experience and foster a trusting patient–provider relationship.

While many therapies for vulvodynia have been used, the following discussion highlights the most common treatment modalities.

Topical

Theoretically, an effective local therapy without the systemic side effects of oral therapies or the risks of surgical treatment would be the ideal therapeutic regimen. Many clinicians will initiate topical therapy for vulvodynia before exploring more invasive options. This is especially true for localized, provoked vulvodynia in which case the most common first line of therapy is topical local anesthetics. While case reports, case series, and retrospective reviews have suggested that topical therapies for vulvodynia may have some efficacy, controlled trials frequently fail to demonstrate a true therapeutic response. However, given the relative safety of topical products, experts in the field of vulvodynia have advocated a trial of topical therapy in the management of women with vulvodynia.

The most common topical therapy used for vulvodynia is local anesthesia. Local anesthetic agents, such as lidocaine and prilocaine, block sodium ion channels and afferent nerve conduction as a result. Given the allodynia noted in the vulvar vestibule in women with vulvodynia, and coupled with the finding of increased innervation in the vestibule of women with localized, provoked vulvodynia, it would seem that a topical anesthetic would effectively decrease pain by inhibiting the afferent signaling of these nerve endings. In one open-label investigation, women with a confirmed diagnosis of localized, provoked vulvodynia were asked to apply 5% lidocaine ointment to the vestibule. After an average of seven weeks of treatment, 76% of women were able to have intercourse as compared to 36% of the cohort before treatment. Additionally, there was a significant decrease in intercourse-related pain scores. However, this study was limited in the lack of a placebo arm. A blinded, randomized controlled trial of topical lidocaine monotherapy as a treatment for localized, provoked vulvodynia was conducted. It was noted that topical lidocaine failed to reduce vulvodynia pain. In fact, subjects in the placebo arm of the study had a

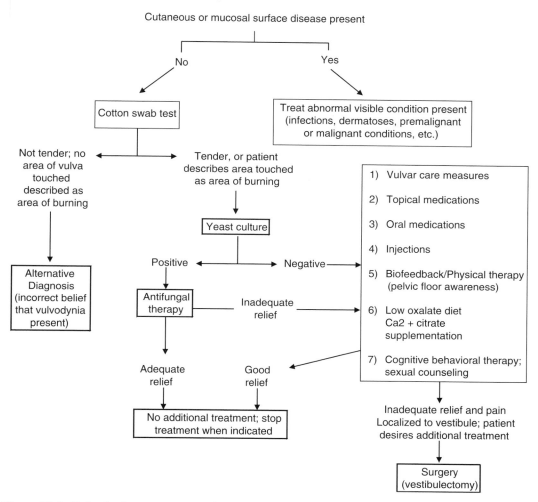

Figure 13.1. Vulvodynia management algorithm. *Adapted from:* Haefner HK, Collins ME, Davis GD, et al. The vulvodynia guideline. *J Lower Gen Tract Dis* 2005; **9**(1): 40–51.

greater improvement than those subjects receiving the active medication, suggesting that there is a strong placebo response, which must be accounted for in investigations of vulvodynia treatment. If vulvodynia truly is a centrally mediated pain syndrome, this may be an explanation for the failure to demonstrate the efficacy of topical local anesthesia.

A number of other topical treatments for vulvodynia have been based on anecdotal evidence and expert opinion. Topical estrogens are commonly used as a treatment for vulvodynia but, in the absence of true atrophic changes, have not

been shown to decrease vulvar pain. Topical nitroglycerin and gabapentin have been reported to result in the clinical improvement in vulvar pain in women with vulvodynia, but only in small open-label studies. Topical corticosteroids, testosterone, and antifungals are generally not effective treatments for vulvodynia.

Injection

Although it is not clear that localized, provoked vulvodynia is a result of vestibular inflammation, there are several reports of various injectable therapies for vulvodynia. Most commonly reported is the infiltration of the vulvar vestibule with a combination of steroid and local anesthetic. These reports have found an improvement in symptoms, but it is important to note that no randomized-controlled trials have been conducted to confirm the effectiveness of this therapy. Case series have suggested that intralesional injection of interferon alpha-2β may result in clinical improvement, but no large-scale investigations have confirmed this finding. While some studies showed some promise in the use of botulinum toxin for the treatment of vulvodynia, blinded, randomized-controlled trials failed to demonstrate superiority of botulinum toxin when compared to placebo in reducing vulvar pain.

Oral

Since vulvodynia is often postulated to be the result of a centrally mediated neuropathic pain syndrome, it would follow that pharmacologic therapies that target the central nervous system might be more effective than topical therapy in alleviating symptoms. Other neuropathic pain syndromes, such as diabetic neuropathy and post-herpetic neuralgia, have effectively been treated with a variety of oral pharmacologic agents that include tricyclic antidepressants, gabapentin, and pregabalin. Although these agents have not been as thoroughly studied for use in treating vulvodynia, they are quite commonly prescribed to treat chronic vulvar pain.

Tricyclic antidepressants

Tricyclic antidepressants, such as amitriptyline, nortriptyline, and desipramine, are used in the treatment of a variety of neuropathic pains, including vulvodynia. This class of medication interacts with 5-HT receptors, increasing serotonin and norepinephrine concentrations in the central nervous system. It is thought that this increase in serotonin potentiates the inhibition of afferent pain signals, thereby resulting in an analgesic effect. Tricyclic antidepressants have anti-cholinergic activity, with the most commonly reported side effects being fatigue and dry mouth. A retrospective review of patients that had had experienced an improvement of symptoms while using amitriptyline for the treatment of vulvodynia found that the average dose in which patients noted some benefit was 40 mg per day, while the average dose for complete symptom resolution was 60 mg per day. Aside from topical xylocaine, the women reviewed in this investigation were using no other therapies. This study found that the patients most likely to respond to amitriptyline were older women, specifically over the age of 40, that had pain described as constant and unremitting. Women with dysparunia seemed less likely to benefit from amitriptyline in this review. Other retrospective reviews have suggested that amitriptyline has efficacy in treatment of vulvodynia, with one reporting a 70% improvement in symptoms and another finding a 90% improvement in symptoms with tricyclic antidepressant use.

⚠ CAUTION! 1

Starting amitriptyline

- Start at a low dose (about 10 mg) and increase slowly to mitigate side effects.
- Use caution when treating elderly women with amitriptyline.
- Caution patients about side effects such as fatigue and dry mouth.

Randomized, controlled trials, however, have yielded more disappointing results than these retrospective reviews of tricyclic antidepressant use for vulvodynia. One randomized controlled trial assessed the use of amitriptyline for generalized and localized vulvodynia, both alone and in combination with a topical steroid. A control group, described as "self management" in this investigation, received no pharmacologic therapy, but did undergo cognitive-behavioral therapy, education, sex therapy, and physical therapy. The investigators found that self-management had a modest effect in reducing vulvar pain symptoms, but management with amitriptyline, both alone and in combination with a topical steroid, was not effective in reducing vulvar pain. Of note, the maximum dose of amitriptyline used in this study was 20 mg per day, well below the average dose where patients noted an effect on symptoms in the previously described retrospective review.

More recently, a randomized, controlled trial assessed the efficacy of two commonly used medical treatments for localized provoked vulvodynia: topical lidocaine monotherapy, oral desipramine (a tricyclic antidepressant) monotherapy, and combined topical lidocaine-oral desipramine. The investigators found that oral desipramine and topical lidocaine, as monotherapy or in combination, failed to reduce vulvodynia pain more than placebo. This investigation again highlights the importance of randomized controlled trials as the basis for designing evidence based treatment protocols, as there seems to be a particularly high placebo effect in vulvodynia treatments. In this investigation, fully 50% of patients in the placebo arm experienced an improvement in symptoms.

Gabapentin

The anticonvulsant gabapentin is a commonly used therapy for neuropathic pain. Though the mechanism of action in treating neuropathic pain is unclear, gabapentin and related compounds (such as pregabalin) mimic the neurotransmitter GABA. Further, gabapentin is thought to interact with voltage gated calcium ion channels and the NDMA receptor. The most commonly reported side effects are dizziness, somnolence, and peripheral edema.

Though gabapentin is very commonly used as a therapy for vulvar pain, there are no randomized, controlled trials demonstrating efficacy for vulvodynia. One case series explored the use of gabapentin in seventeen women with chronic unexplained vulvar pain. Patients initiated gabapentin at a dose of 300 mg, and this dose was increased until patients experienced relief of symptoms or a maximum dose of 1200 mg was achieved. The authors of this small study reported that 82% of patients had either complete or partial relief of symptoms, with more than half of patients reporting side effects (headaches, nausea, vomiting, fatigue and dizziness). Another retrospective investigation of gabapentin use for vulvodynia found that the medication was well tolerated, and that 64% of patients had resolution of at least 80% of their symptoms during the study. Gabapentin remains a reasonable option for managing patients with vulvodynia. However, more rigorous study is needed to say with certainty that gabapentin has efficacy in treating vulvodynia.

Other oral agents

Pregabalin and selective-serotonin reuptake inhibitors are other oral agents used to treat vulvodynia.

Vestibulectomy

For most clinicians, surgical management of vulvodynia is considered as a last resort. The prospect of undergoing surgery with the potential for permanent changes in the appearance of the vulva is understandably daunting for patients. The clinician must also carefully consider the subtype of vulvodynia from which the patient is suffering. As most surgical procedures for vulvodynia are directed at removing all or a portion of the vestibule, many women experiencing pain in other regions of the vulva more consistent with generalized vulvodynia would be suboptimally treated with removal of the vestibule. The decision to proceed with surgical therapy therefore requires a careful history and physical examination, with particular attention to the precise areas of the vulva where the patient is experiencing pain. Further, the patient should be thoroughly counseled as to the risks and benefits of surgical management. In the properly selected patient with localized vulvodynia however, the surgical management of vulvodynia may be an excellent choice.

✋ CAUTION! 2

Vestibulectomy
Hematoma formation is not uncommon following vestibulectomy. Be sure to cauterize any bleeding vessels during the procedure. After closure, inspect the vulva for any signs of hematoma formation. Advise the patient to monitor for development increasing pain or development of a mass at the incision.

The most common surgical therapy for vulvodynia is *vestibulectomy*. Various techniques for the procedure have been described. Initial descriptions of vestibulectomy advocated the removal of the entire vestibule of the vagina. Recognizing that many patients with localized, provoked vulvodynia have symptoms isolated to posterior vestibule, the procedure has been subsequently modified such that only the posterior vestibule is removed. Removing only the posterior vestibule diminishes the risk of injuring the urethra, but could result in persistent symptoms if the patient is suffering from anterior vestibular pain.

When performing the typical modified vestibulectomy (Table 13.2), the area of vulvar pain should be initially mapped with a marking pen while the patient is awake. Generally, the procedure is carried out under general or regional anesthesia, though in the properly selected patient local anesthesia may be a reasonable choice. In many cases, the area of excision will include the vestibule from 3 o'clock to 9 o'clock, but may need to extend anteriorly as far as the peri-urethral region, depending on the location of the patient's pain. The vestibule can be infiltrated with local anesthesia in the area to be excised, with or without a vasopressive agent such as epinephrine. The vestibule is then excised to a depth of 2–3 mm in a "U-shape" with the hymeneal ring being the proximal margin and Hart's line being the distal margin. The vaginal mucosa can be undermined to a distance of 1–2 cm, thereby freeing the mucosa of tension as it is attached to the perineal skin. A variety of closure techniques can be used, but this author favors closure in two layers with the superficial layer closed with interrupted vertical mattress sutures.

Table 13.2. Steps for performing vestibulectomy

---

1. Before the patient receives anesthesia, use a marking pen to mark all of the areas of the vestibule that are painful for the patient.

2. Infiltrate the area to be excised with a local anesthesia, with or without a vasopressive agent.

3. Excise the marked area using the hymeneal ring as the proximal margin and Hart's line as the distal margin.

4. Undermine 1–2 cm of the vaginal mucosa using scissors or the electrosurgical instrument.

5. Close the wound in two layers. For the superficial layer, use vertical mattress sutures.

While vestibulectomy is generally a surgery with low morbidity, the procedure is not without risk. Hemorrhage and hematoma formation can occur following vestibulectomy, with reported incidence of 1% to 6.2%. Additionally, surgical site infection occurs about 1% of the time following vestibulectomy. Other complications following vestibulectomy include scarring, decreased lubrication, and Bartholin's gland cyst formation.

The weight of evidence suggests that vestibulectomy is an efficacious therapy for localized provoked vulvodynia. Reported success rates for vestibulectomy range between 70% and 100%, with success variably defined as improvement of dysparunia, increased sexual function, and decreased vestibular tenderness. Patients must be counseled, however, that recovery from vestibulectomy is an extended process. Physical therapy may be necessary after the incision has healed to facilitate the patient's recovery and to prepare for attempted intercourse. Further, patients must be counseled that not everyone will improve following vestibulectomy.

Laser

Laser therapy has demonstrated efficacy for the treatment of several vulvar conditions, including vulvar intraepithelial neoplasia (VIN) and condyloma accuminatum. However, laser therapy has not proven to be an effective strategy for treating vulvodynia, and as such should be avoided.

Physical therapy

Pelvic floor physical therapy is an important adjunct to any comprehensive management plan for women with vulvodynia. Women with vulvodynia that complete a physical therapy program are likely to experience symptom reduction, an improvement in sexual function, and an increased quality of life. Women with both generalized and localized vulvodynia benefit from physical therapy. Physical therapy is especially useful in women with vaginismus, a condition characterized by painful, involuntary spasm of the muscles surrounding the outer vagina. The variety of techniques employed by physical therapists in treating vulvodynia are outlined in Table 13.3.

It is of particular importance that the patient establishes care with a physical therapist with

Table 13.3. Physical therapy techniques

Internal and external soft tissue mobilization and myofascial release

Trigger point pressure

Visceral, urogenital, and joint manipulation

Electrical stimulation

Therapeutic exercises

Active pelvic floor retraining

Biofeedback

Bladder and bowel retraining

Therapeutic ultrasound

Home vaginal dilation

expertise in treating women with vulvodynia. Physical therapy for vulvodynia is quite invasive and can be uncomfortable, especially for women already suffering from vulvar pain. Special training in vulvar physical therapy techniques, and a thorough understanding of the disease process, are imperative.

Acupuncture

Though acupuncture has been shown to be remarkably effective for a variety of pain syndromes, two studies of acupuncture for the treatment of vulvodynia have drawn less promising conclusions. One small study reported the experience of 12 patients that underwent acupuncture for vulvodynia, with only two patients reporting themselves "cured" and seven patients feeling only slightly better or not better at all. Similarly, another study found no significantly increased ability for eight women with vulvodynia to have intercourse after completing treatment with acupuncture, though there was some reduction in pain with manual genital stimulation.

Conclusion

Vulvodynia is a fairly common syndrome of uncertain etiology. The patient presenting with chronic vulvar pain should have a thorough medical history and physical examination to insure that an accurate diagnosis is made. Treatments for vulvodynia remain suboptimal, but a comprehensive management pain can result in a reduction in symptoms and improved quality of life. Randomized-controlled trials are needed to establish effective evidence-based management strategies.

Bibliography

Arnold LG, Bachmann GA, Rosen R. Vulvodynia: characteristics and associations with co-morbidities and quality of life. *Obstet Gynecol* 2006; **107**(3): 617–624.

Ben-David B, Friedman M. Gabapentin therapy for vulvodynia. *Anesth Analg* 1999; **89**(6): 1459–1460.

Brown CS, Wan J, Bachmann G, et al. Self-management, amitriptyline, and amitriptyline plus triamcinolone in the management of vulvodynia. *J Womens Health (Larchmt)* 2009; **18**(2): 163–169.

Chadha S, Gianotten WL, Drogendijk AC. Histopathologic features of vulvar vestibulitis. *Int J Gynecol Pathol* 1998; **17**(1): 7–11.

Curran S, Brotto LA, Fisher H, et al. The ACTIV study: acupuncture treatment in provoked vestibulodynia. *J Sex Med* 2010; **7**(2 pt 2): 981–995.

Eva LJ, Rolfe KJ, MacLean AB. Is localized, provoked vulvodynia an inflammatory condition? *J Repro Med* 2007; **52**(5): 379–384.

Foster DC, Kotok MB, Huang L.S. et al. Oral desipramine and topical lidocaine for vulvodynia: a randomized, controlled trial. *Obstet Gynecol* 2010; **116**(3): 583–593.

Giesecke J, Reed BD, Haefner HK, et al. Quantitative sensory testing in vulvodynia patients and increased peripheral pain sensitivity 2004; **104**(1): 125–133.

Harlow BL, Stewart EG. A population-based assessment of chronic unexplained vulvar pain: have we underestimated the prevalence of vulvodynia? *J Am Meds Womens Assoc* 2003; **58**(2): 82–88.

Harlow BL, Stewart EG. Adult-onset vulvodynia in relation to childhood violence victimization. *Am J Epidemiol* 2005; **9**: 871–880.

Harris G, Horowitz B, Borgida A. Evaluation of gabapentin in the treatment of generalized vulvodynia, unprovoked. *J Repro Med* 2007; **52**(2): 103–106.

Masheb RM, Wang E, Lozano C, et al. Prevalence and correlates of depression in treatment-seeking women with vulvodynia. *J Obstet Gynaecol* 2005; **25**(8): 786–791.

McCay M. Dysesthetic ("essential") vulvodynia. Treatment with amitriptyline. *J Repro Med* 1993; **38**(1): 9–13.

Munday PE. Response to treatment in dysaesthetic vulvodynia. *J Obstet Gynaecol* 2001; **21**(6): 610–613.

Petersen CD, Giraldi A, Lundvall L. et al. Botulinum toxin type A – a novel treatment for provoked vestibulodynia? Results of a randomized, placebo controlled, double-blinded study. *J Sex Med* 2009; **9**: 2523–2537.

Ponte M, Klemperer E, Sahay A, et al. Effects of vulvodynia on quality of life. *J Am Acad Dermatol* 2009; **60**(1): 70–76.

Powell J, Wojnarowska F. Acupuncture for vulvodynia. *J R Soc Med* 1999; **92**(11): 579–581.

Reed BD, Haefner HK, Sen A, et al. Vulvodynia incidence and remission rates among adult women: a 2 year follow up study. *Obstet Gynecol* 2008; **112**(2 part 1): 231–237.

Reed BD, Caron AM, Gorenflo DW, et al. Treatment of vulvodynia with tricyclic antidepressants: efficacy and associated factors. *J Low Genit Tract Dis* 2006; **10**(4): 245–251.

Reed BD, Haefner HK, Punch MR, et al. Psychosocial and sexual functioning in women with vulvodynia and chronic pelvic pain. A comparative evaluation. *J Repro Med* 2000; **45**(8): 624–632.

Schmidt S, Bauer A, Grief C, et al. Vulvar Pain. *Psychol Prof Treat Resp* 2001; **46**(4): 377–384.

Tommola P, Unkila-Kallio L, Paavonen J. Surgical treatment of vulvar vestibulitis: a review. *Acta Obstet Gynecol Scan* 2010; **89**(11): 1385–1395.

Updike GM, Wiesenfeld HC. Insights into the management of vulvar pain: a survey of clinicians. *Am J Obstet Gynecol* 2005; **193**(4): 1404–1409.

Zolnoun DA, Hartmann KE, Steege JF. Overnight 5% lidocaine ointment for treatment of vulvar vestibulitis 2003; **102**(1): 84–87.

Vulvar Cancer

Ashlee Smith and Kristin K. Zorn

Department of Obstetrics, Gynecology & Reproductive Sciences, Division of Reproductive Infectious Diseases, Magee-Womens Hospital of the University of Pittsburgh Medical Center, Pittsburgh, PA, USA

Introduction

Vulvar cancer is the fourth most common gynecologic cancer and comprises 5% of malignancies of the female genital tract. Presentations of vulvar cancer can often mimic other benign gynecologic conditions, including genital ulcer disease (of either infectious or noninfectious etiology), or occur in a background of chronic vulvar inflammatory conditions. This fact often predisposes to misdiagnosis and/or delayed diagnosis, thus affecting prognosis. Knowledge of these overlapping presentations may help to lessen the overall burden of disease from vulvar cancer. Annually, there are an estimated 3,580 new cases and 900 deaths from this disease in the United States. Squamous cell carcinomas account for approximately 90% of cases, whereas melanoma (5–10%), basal cell carcinoma (2%), and sarcoma (1–2%), and extramammary Paget's disease (2%) are much less common. Paget's disease of the vulva is an intraepithelial neoplasm arising as an aberrant differentiation of apocrine glandular cells. The diagnosis and treatment are often confusing and complex. Underlying invasive malignancy can be found in approximately 10–20% of patients affected by this disorder. Although the rate of invasive vulvar cancer has remained stable during the past two decades, the rate of in situ disease has more than doubled. Recent research has been aimed at better understanding the natural progression of the disease, prevention, earlier detection, and less morbid treatments.

Epidemiology

A key historical distinguishing feature of vulvar cancer from other benign vulvar conditions is that it tends to occur in post-menopausal women, with the peak incidence between 65 and 75 years old. There is no predilection for a specific race or culture; gravidity and parity are not associated with its pathogenesis. Risk factors for vulvar cancer include cigarette smoking, vulvar dystrophy, vulvar or cervical intraepithelial neoplasia, human papillomavirus (HPV) infection, immunodeficiency syndromes, and a prior history of cervical cancer. Unfortunately, however, the number of young women with invasive disease appears to be increasing.

> ★ **TIPS & TRICKS**
>
> - Vulvar cancer has a bimodal age distribution.
> - Risk factors for vulvar cancer: smoking, vulvar dystrophy, VIN, HPV, immunodeficiency, prior cervical cancer

As these risk factors suggest, two independent pathways of vulvar carcinogenesis are felt to exist,

---

one related to chronic inflammation and auto-immune processes and the second related to mucosal HPV infection. Invasive cancer is often seen in association with preinvasive disease in younger women, whereas the elderly patients often do not have VIN but rather a background of lichen sclerosus. This suggests that the inflammation pathway is often the source of vulvar cancer in older women, while younger women tend to develop HPV-associated vulvar dysplasia and cancer.

HPV is a double-stranded DNA virus shown to be responsible for 60% of vulvar cancers. Increasing rates of vulvar intraepithelial neoplasia (VIN) have been associated with HPV infection and related to changing sexual behavior, HPV infection, and cigarette smoking. The estimated prevalence of anogenital tract HPV infections within the United States is 20 million, with an annual incidence of 5.5 million cases. It has been estimated that 75 to 80% of sexually active adults will acquire a genital tract HPV infection before the age of 50. Many sexually active young women have sequential infections with different oncogenic types of HPV. These infections are frequently transient and often produce reversible cytologic changes.

Different oncogenic types of HPV have a propensity to infect varying body sites. HPV strains with a predilection for infection of mucous membranes often result in infections of the penis, scrotum, perineum, perianal region, vaginal introitus, vulva, and cervix. Condylomata acuminata are benign anogenital warts, most often caused by HPV types 6 and 11. A relationship has been documented between HPV types 16 and 18 and intraepithelial neoplasia of the vulva, vagina, penis, anus, and cervix (Table 14.1). These subtypes have also been linked to carcinomas of the same areas.

The transmission of HPV is related to close personal contact. The most common predictor of genital HPV infection has been sexual activity. The risk of HPV infection in women is directly related to the number of male sex partners and to the male partners' number of female sex partners. Sex with a new partner is a stronger risk factor than sex with a steady partner. Vaginal or anal intercourse is a major risk factor for HPV infection, although penetrating vaginal intercourse is not required.

Table 14.1. HPV types and estimates of disease burden

HPV type	Approximate disease burden
16 and 18	■ 70% of cervical cancer, AIS, CIN 3, VIN 2/3, and VaIN 2/3 cases
	■ 50% of CIN 2 cases
6, 11, 16, and 18	■ 35%–50% of all CIN 1, VIN 1, and VaIN 1 cases
	■ 90% of genital warts cases

AIS: adenocarcinoma in situ; CIN: Cervical intraepithelial neoplasia; VIN: vulvar intraepithelial neoplasia; VaIN: vaginal intraepithelial neoplasia

Two vaccines have been developed against HPV infection. A quadrivalent vaccine (Gardasil™) targets HPV types 16 and 18, which cause approximately 70% of cervical cancers and about 50% of pre-cancerous lesions, as well as types 6 and 11, which cause 90% of genital warts. The vaccine is administered in three doses at time 0, 2, and 6 months. Cervarix™ is a bivalent vaccine that targets HPV types 16 and 18. This vaccine is given in three doses at time 0, 1, and 6 months. Presently, studies of cervical dysplasia have shown that administration of the quadrivalent vaccine is 98% effective in preventing the development of CIN II, III, or adenocarcinoma in situ related to the acquisition of HPV types 16 and 18. In the Future I study, Gardasil™ had 100% efficacy in preventing external anogenital and vaginal lesions related to HPV subtypes 6, 11, 16, and 18.

★ TIPS &TRICKS

- HPV subtypes 16 and 18 are linked to the development of vulvar dysplasia and cancer, while 6 and 11 cause genital warts.
- Persistent, confluent genital warts should be biopsied liberally to rule out malignancy.
- Bivalent and quadrivalent vaccines are currently available to help prevent HPV acquisition.

Table 14.2. Guidelines for HPV vaccination

Recommendations	ACIP	ACOG	AAFP	AAP
Routine vaccination in females 11–12 years old and catch-up vaccination in 13-to 26-year-olds	Y	Y	Y	Y
Females 9–10 years old can be vaccinated	Y	Y	Y	Y
Vaccinate regardless of previous HPV infection or abnormal Pap test results	Y	Y	Y	Y
Continue Pap testing after vaccination	Y	Y	Y	Y

ACIP: Advisory Committee on Immunization Practices; ACOG: American College of Obstetricians and Gynecologists; AAFP: American Academy of Family Physicians; AAP: American Academy of Pediatrics

Although Gardasil™ was initially approved for the prevention of cervical cancer, the indications have broadened to also include the prevention of vaginal and vulvar dysplasia based on the findings from the Future I and II study results. At this time, there is no comparable data for the bivalent vaccine as vulvar and vaginal dysplasia endpoints were not assessed in those studies.

Guidelines for the administration of the vaccine vary between committees (Table 14.2). The Advisory Committee on Immunization Practices (ACIP) and the American College of Obstetricians and Gynecologists (ACOG) recommend HPV vaccination administration between from 9 to –26 years in girls and women who have not been previously vaccinated. Catch-up vaccination is supported by both groups and neither endorses a preference between the two types of vaccine.

The American Cancer Society (ACS) guidelines recommend the HPV vaccine be routinely offered between the ages of 11 and 18 years, with no catch-up vaccination for women 19–26 years. Currently, the ACIP also supports the administration of the quadrivalent vaccine to males aged 9–26.

It should be stressed that although HPV vaccination holds great promise for future vulvar, vaginal, and cervical cancer prevention, it is a prophylactic rather than a therapeutic strategy. As such, the presence or absence of HPV vaccination has no bearing on the management of current genital lesions.

Clinical evaluation and staging

Most patients present with a vulvar lump or mass, often with a history of pruritis, especially if the lesion appears in the setting of vulvar dystrophy. Long-term pruritis or a lump or mass in the vagina is present in >50% of patients with invasive vulvar cancer. Other symptoms could include pain, ulceration, vaginal bleeding, discharge, or dysuria. It is important to note that all of these symptoms are frequent complaints among women, which suggest an infectious etiology, and are often treated as such. Occasionally, women may present with a large mass in the groin which is representative of metastasis to the lymph nodes.

In reported series of vulvar carcinoma, a 2- to 16-month delay is common in patients seeking medical treatment. Further, medical treatment of vulvar lesions often continues for up to 12 months or longer without adequate visual inspection, biopsy, or referral. Physician delay remains a common problem in the diagnosis of vulvar cancer. In young patients, this delay is often associated with a wart appearance presumed to be benign (Figure 14.1).

Although isolated condylomata do not require a histologic diagnosis, any confluent warty lesion should be biopsied adequately before medical or ablative therapy is initiated. Older patients and the physician may both be reluctant to insist on a thorough pelvic examination, preferring instead to treat vulvar symptoms as a presumed case of yeast infection, urinary infection, or post-menopausal atrophy. While those issues certainly should be considered in the differential diagnosis, only a full inspection with biopsies of suspicious lesions can establish the correct diagnosis. This may require an examination under anesthesia

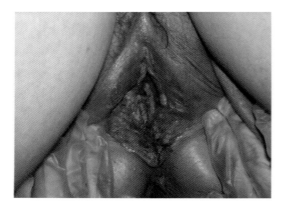

Figure 14.1. A 33-year-old woman with a longstanding history of genital warts. Biopsy was deferred as the clinician was confident this was "just warts." Patient was ultimately diagnosed with advanced vulvar cancer, which led to her death despite aggressive chemoradiation.

with liberal biopsies of suspicious lesions, especially those that do not respond to standard therapies for benign conditions. Fortunately, vulvar cancer is commonly indolent, extends slowly, and metastasizes relatively late in the disease course. This progression allows physicians and healthcare providers the opportunity to make a diagnosis before the disease spreads. Patient awareness, education, and thorough annual examination offer several opportunities to limit or prevent advanced disease.

Physical examination often reveals raised or flat lesions which may be fleshy, ulcerated, leukoplakic, or warty. Biopsy must be completed on all suspicious lesions of the vulva, including lumps, ulcers, and pigmented areas, regardless of patient complaints or symptoms. The biopsy specimen must include some underlying dermis and connective tissue so that the pathologist can adequately determine the depth and nature of a stromal invasion.

> **★ TIPS & TRICKS**
>
> - Vulvar cancer develops slowly, providing ample opportunity for early diagnosis.
> - Early stage disease is highly treatable and curable.

> - Biopsy all suspicious lesions including lumps, ulcers, pigmented areas, especially when not responsive to traditional therapies.
> - Cancerous lesions may not be symptomatic, making annual vulvar inspection a must.

A complete pelvic and physical examination is performed, with particular attention to the measurement of the diameter of the primary tumor and palpation for inguinal, axillary, or supraclavicular lymphadenopathy. A Pap smear should be taken from the cervix, and a colposcopy of the cervix and vagina should be performed because of the common association with other squamous intraepithelial neoplasms. For women with large tumors or suspected metastases, an abdominal/pelvic computed tomography may be performed to evaluate for lymphadenopathy or other metastases.

Table 14.3 describes the standard surgical staging system adopted and utilized by the International Federation of Gynecology and Obstetrics, derived from primary tumor characteristics (size and depth of invasion), regional lymph nodes, and distant metastasis.

Anatomy/pattern of spread

Although disease can occur anywhere on the vulva, approximately 70% of cancers arise primarily on the labia. Vulvar cancer spreads by:

1. Direct extension, to involve adjacent organs and structures.
2. Lymphatic embolization to regional lymph nodes.
3. Hematogenous dissemination to affect distant sites such as the lungs, liver, and bone.

The primary route of lymphatic spread is by way of the superficial inguinal, deep femoral (located beneath the cribiform fascia), and external iliac lymph nodes. The Cloquet node, the last node in the femoral chain, is located just beneath the Poupart ligament and is noted to be absent in approximately 54% of specimens dissected. Most experts agree that the superficial inguinal lymph nodes are the primary nodal group for the vulva and can therefore serve as the sentinel nodes for

Table 14.3. FIGO staging for vulvar carcinoma (revised 2009)

Stage I	Tumor confined to the vulva	
	IA	Lesions ≤2 cm in size, confined to the vulva or perineum and with stromal invasion ≤1.0 mm, no nodal metastasis
	IB	Lesions >2 cm in size or with stromal invasion >1.0 mm, confined to the vulva or perineum, with negative nodes
Stage II	Tumor of any size with extension to adjacent perineal structures (lower 1/3 urethra, lower 1/3 vagina, anus) with negative nodes	
Stage III	Tumor of any size with or without extension to adjacent perineal structures (lower 1/3 urethra, lower 1/3 vagina, anus)	with positive inguino-femoral lymph nodes
	IIIA	(i) With 1 lymph node metastasis (≥ 5 mm), or (ii) 1–2 lymph node metastasis(es) (<5 mm)
	IIIB	(i) With 2 or more lymph node metastasis (≥5 mm), or (ii) 3 or more lymph node metastasis (<5 mm)
	IIIC	With positive nodes with extracapsular spread
Stage IV	Tumor invades other regional (upper 2/3 urethra, upper 2/3 vagina) or distant structures	
	IVA	Tumor invades any of the following: (i) upper urethra and or vaginal mucosa, bladder mucosa, rectal mucosa, or fixed to the pelvic bone, or (ii) fixed or ulcerated inguino-femoral lymph nodes
	IVB	Any distant metastasis including pelvic lymph nodes

this region. Contralateral spread may result from the rich intercommunicating lymphatic system of the vulva. Lateralized lesions generally spread to the ipsilateral groin. Midline lesions, or lesions less than 1 cm from the midline, can drain to either side. Although lymphatics from the clitoris directly to the deep pelvic lymph nodes are described, their clinical significance appears to be minimal. Lymphatic drainage of the vulva is a progressive systematic mechanism allowing therapy to be planned according to where in the lymph node chain tumor is present.

Treatment

The treatment of vulvar dysplasia depends to some extent on the symptoms of the patient and the associated pathology. Outside of patients in immune-compromised states, heavy smokers, and the elderly, the progression of early dysplastic lesions to carcinoma in situ or cancer is slow, and for some patients never occurs. In young women, persistence of disease or spontaneous regression can occur, especially when linked to multifocal lesions and HPV-dependent disease. However, it is important to remember the possibility of an occult underlying invasive lesion. The frequency of this event varies by the population studies and the degree of dysplasia. Importantly, it is reported that up to 22% of vulvar carcinoma in situ lesions (also known as VIN 3) undergoing resection have an underlying malignancy on the final pathologic review.

During the 1980s, the treatment paradigms for vulvar cancer began to shift. Historically, all patients with vulvar cancer were staged and treated surgically with a radical total vulvectomy and an en bloc inguinofemoral lymph node dissection. This procedure was associated with high rates of survival, but also with high rates of morbidity. Current approaches individualize treatment so that the most conservative procedure is used to optimize patient survival and minimize perioperative morbidity.

Less radical surgeries were described and combined with chemotherapy, radiation, or both. Using groin incisions that are separate from the vulvar incision dramatically decreased the rates of wound infection, while radical groin dissections were omitted from routine practice in patients with superficial, early-stage disease.

There is currently, a standard radical vulvectomy with dissection completed to the urogenital diaphragm and tumor-free margins of at least 1–2 cm. Inguinofemoral lymphadenectomy is performed for all stages of disease except stage IA. Bilateral lymphadenectomy is performed for stage II or greater disease, central stage IB disease (<1 cm from the vulvar midline), or if lymph node metastases are discovered with the ipsilateral groin dissection.

Sentinel lymph node mapping, originally developed in the management of breast cancer and melanoma, has become a viable option for the evaluation of groin metastases in early vulvar cancer. New information about the natural variation in lymphatic drainage from the primary site has been gathered via lymphatic mapping techniques. The purpose of mapping is to identify a sentinel node or nodal group that serves as the initial drainage site for the primary lesion. These nodes are at highest risk for metastasis and should be representative of nodal pathology for the entire groin. The procedure is currently being performed with vital blue dye, lymphoscintigraphy, or both. A negative sentinel lymph node evaluation could reduce the need for complete groin dissection and eliminate the morbidity associated with the extensive dissection.

When tumor involves the urethra, anus, or is too bulky for surgical resection, chemoradiation has become the therapy of choice. While the specifics of chemoradiation in vulvar cancer will not be addressed in this review, the improvement in survival and decreased morbidity seen in the population of vulvar cancer patients with advanced disease echoes the success seen with patients with earlier stages of disease.

Protocols for follow-up after primary and adjuvant therapy vary from institution to institution. Close surveillance and follow-up is nearly always recommended for the first 2–3 years. With this surveillance, more than 75% of recurrences are detected. Given the potential for a field effect with both chronic inflammation and HPV infection, the two precursor lesions know to predispose to vulvar cancer, the vagina, vulva, and cervix of women with a prior diagnosis of vulvar cancer remain at risk for further dysplasia and malignancy.

Prognosis

The principal prognostic factors related to cancers of the vulva are the presence or absence of regional lymph node metastasis, size and location of the lesion, and histologic subtype. In the early part of the 20th century, patients commonly presented with advanced disease, during a time period when surgical techniques were poorly developed. Therefore, the initial 5-year survival rates for vulvar cancer were 20–25%. Today, with stage I and II disease, the corrected 5-year survival rate is greater than 90%. A 75% corrected 5-year survival rate for all stages of vulvar cancer is reported by most institutions. Patients with positive nodes have been noted to experience recurrence earlier than patients with negative nodes. Bilateral lymph node involvement has a more ominous prognosis that unilateral lymph node involvement. Not surprisingly, local relapse is associated with positive or close surgical margins, capillary space involvement, greater depth of invasion, and a large primary lesion size.

Recurrent vulvar cancer is an ominous finding. However, the possibility also exists for a second primary tumor, rather than a true recurrence of the original tumor. Prognosis largely depends on whether the new lesion occurs in a previously treated field. Locally recurrent vulvar cancer occasionally can be excised. In the setting of previous vulvar radiation, wound breakdown becomes a serious morbidity. Radical surgery, such as an exenteration or a modified exenterative procedure, is sometimes indicated as the only attempt for cure or symptom relief. Limited data on exenteration procedures for recurrent disease has suggested an approximate 38% 5-year survival.

Summary

Vulvar cancer is a relatively rare gynecologic cancer which tends to be associated with precursor lesions. In young women, HPV infection causes genital warts, which, when persistent, can lead to VIN and vulvar cancer. In older women, chronic inflammatory conditions such as lichen sclerosus may lead to vulvar cancer without associated VIN. Surveillance of women with pre-cancerous conditions, careful examination of vulvar lesions, and early biopsy of suspicious lesions are the cornerstones of effective management. Attention to the often overlapping clinical presentation of infectious genital ulcers, other STI-related complaints, and vulvar neoplasms is warranted. These principles should help to reduce the rate of advanced vulvar cancer now, while the introduction of widespread HPV vaccination may help to prevent vulvar cancer in the future.

Bibliography

Advisory Committee on Immunization Practices. Recommended adult immunization schedule: United States, 2010. *Ann Inter Med* 2010; **152**: 36.

American College of Obstetricians and Gynecologists. ACOG Practice Bulletin Clinical Management Guidelines for Obstetricians–Gynecologists. Number 61, April 2005. Human Papillomavirus. *Obstet Gynecol* 2005; **105**: 905.

Berek JS, Hacker NF. *Gynecologic Oncology*, 5th edn. Lippincott Williams & Wilkins, 2009.

Beutner KR. Nongenital human papillomavirus infections. *Clin Lab Med* 2000; **20**: 423.

Bodelon C, Madeline MM, Voigt LF, Weiss NS. Is the incidence of vulvar cancer increasing in the United States? *Cancer Causes Control* 2009; **20**: 1779.

Center for Disease Control and Prevention, Workowski KA, Berman SM. Sexually transmitted diseases treatment guidelines, 2006. *MMWR Recomm Rep* 2006; **55**: 1.

DiSaia PJ, Creaseman WT. *Clinical Gynecologic Oncology*, 7th edn. Elsevier Health Sciences, 2007.

Dunne EF, Unger ER, Sternberg M, et al. Prevalence of HPV infection among females in the United States. *J Am Med Assoc* 2007; **297**: 813.

FUTURE II Study Group. Quadrivalent vaccine against human papillomavirus to prevent high-grade cervical lesions. *New Engl J Med* 2007; **356**: 1915.

Gonzalez Bosquet J, Magrina JF, Magtibay PM, et al. Patterns of inguinal groin metastases in squamous cell carcinoma of the vulva. *Gynecol Oncol* 2007; **105**: 742.

Hampl M, Deckers-Figiel S, Hampl JA, et al. New aspects of vulvar cancer: changes in localization and age of onset. *Gynecol Oncol* 2008; **109**: 340.

Jemal A, Siegel R, Xu J, Ward E. Cancer statistics, 2010. *CA Cancer J Clin* 2010; **60**: 277.

Jones RW, Rowan DM, Stewart AW. Vulvar intraepithelial neoplasia. Aspects of the natural history and outcome in 405 women. *Obstet Gynecol* 2005; **106**: 1319.

Levenback C, Coleman RL, Burke TW, et al. Intraoperative lymphatic mapping and sentinel node identification with blue dye in patients with vulvar cancer. *Gynecol Oncol* 2001; **83**: 276.

McCormack PL, Joura EA. Quadrivalent human papillomavirus (Types 6, 11, 16, 18) recombinant vaccine (Gardasil®). *Drugs* 2010; **70**: 2449.

Peyton CL, Gravitt PE, Hunt WC, et al. Determinants of genital human papillomavirus detection in a US population. *J Infect Dis* 2001; **183**: 1154.

Winer RL, Lee SK, Hughes JP, et al. Genital human papillomavirus infection: incidence and risk factors in a cohort of female university students. *Am J Epidemiol* 2003; **157**: 218.

Different Manifestations and Implications of Sexually Transmitted Infections and Vagnitides in Pregnancy

Noor Niyar N. Ladhani and Mark H. Yudin

Department of Obstetrics and Gynecology, University of Toronto, and St. Michael's Hospital, Toronto, Canada

Introduction

Sexually transmitted infections and vaginitides during pregnancy can have adverse effects on the health of the mother, the developing fetus, and the newborn child. Transmission in utero can impact embryogenesis and development, while vertical transmission during delivery can cause early disease processes in the vulnerable infant. In addition, evidence is increasing to suggest a link between the inflammatory environment caused by these infectious processes and adverse pregnancy outcomes such as preterm labor, preterm premature rupture of membranes, and low birth weight infants.

The maternal effects of these conditions have great public health importance unto themselves. The burden of disease is multiplied when considering the short- and long-term effects they have on the offspring. Some of these last well into adulthood and can cause significant developmental and physical morbidity. A good understanding of these processes and how they must be treated is important in the prevention of these avoidable consequences.

Sexually transmitted infections

Sexually transmitted infections (STIs) are common world wide. There are similar risk factors for many of these infections, including young age, previous STI, new or multiple sex partners, inconsistent condom use, sex work, and illicit drug use. Treatment in pregnancy is imperative to prevent the spread of the disease to other sexual partners as well as to prevent transmission to the fetus and the newborn. The presentation and implications of several common STIs are discussed in this chapter. HIV and the hepatitides are outside the scope of the chapter, but their management in pregnancy requires the care of a multidisciplinary team specializing in the management of these complex cases.

Chlamydia

Clinical characteristics

The various serovars of *Chlamydia trachomatis* are responsible for urogenital infections, lymphgranuloma venereum, and ocular trachoma. Genital infections with *C. trachomatis* are the most commonly reported infectious disease in

---

Sexually Transmitted Diseases, First Edition. Edited by Richard H. Beigi.

North America and the most common bacterial STI world wide. Among couples in which one partner is infected, sexual transmission to the other partner has been reported to be as high as 75% world wide, and infection rates in pregnancy range from 1.9% up to 26%, depending on geographic region and population characteristics.

> ⚕ **CAUTION!**
>
> Chlamydia is the most common bacterial STI world wide. Screening based on risk factors misses at least a third of infections, so all women should be screened in pregnancy. Because reinfection rates are high, repeat screening in the third trimester should also be considered.

Most cases in women are asymptomatic, and detection by screening these asymptomatic women is important. Rescreening high-risk individuals in the third trimester is necessary, even when an infection has been treated early in pregnancy and test of cure has been proven. When present, clinical features of urogenital infection include vaginal discharge, mucopurulent cervical discharge, contact or postcoital bleeding, dysuria, and urethritis.

Maternal and fetal effects

Vertical transmission of chlamydia poses the greatest risk to the newborn. Conflicting evidence also exists for the impact of recent infection on rates of adverse pregnancy outcomes such as preterm birth and low birth weight infants. Infection can impact maternal health by causing postpartum endometritis as well as future infertility and subfertility.

> ♺ **SCIENCE REVISITED**
>
> The role of chlamydia infection in causing adverse pregnancy outcomes: The infectious agent has been recovered from amniotic fluid and from placenta, and may have a role in causing stillbirths. Preterm

---

labor and preterm premature rupture of membranes have also been shown to be increased with the presence of *C. trachomatis* infection or serologic evidence of infection, and may be due to a subclinical chorioamnionitis or by the immunologic reaction triggered by the presence of infection. Delivery of a low birth weight infant has been shown to be associated with *C. trachomatis* infection, especially among term cases, but such an association has also not been identified in several cohort studies. In vitro studies have implicated *C. trachomatis* in intrauterine growth restriction cases through placental apoptosis when chronic infection is present.

Transmission rates from infected, untreated mothers to neonates at the time of childbirth can be as high at 50–75%. Transmission usually occurs during vaginal birth but has also been seen in Caesarean deliveries with intact membranes. Twenty to fifty percent of infected infants develop conjunctivitis and 5–20% develop pneumonia. Asymptomatic infections of the mucous membranes of the newborn's eye, oropharynx, urogenital tract, and rectum may also occur.

Conjunctivitis usually appears at 5 to 12 days of life, though any conjunctivitis occurring at less than 30 days of life should raise suspicion for a *C. trachomatis* ophthalmia neonatorum. Conjunctival exudate and cells should be swabbed and sent for culture or nonculture testing. *Neisseria gonorrhoeae* should be excluded, though this form of ophthalmia neonatorum usually presents earlier. If diagnosed, the newborn, the mother, and her sex partners should be treated.

Chlamydia trachomatis pneumonia should be considered in all infants less than 3 months of age who present with a suspicious clinical picture. A repetitive staccato cough and tachypnea, as well as chest radiographs showing hyperinflation of the lungs and bilateral diffuse infiltrates, are suggestive of this pneumonia. The infants usually look well, are afebrile, and do not wheeze. Swabs of nasopharynx should be sent for tissue culture to confirm the diagnosis but, if this is suspected, the initiation of empiric treatment should be considered.

Diagnosis (in the mother)

Specimens for urogenital chlamydia infections can be obtained from urine samples and endocervical or vaginal swabs. Generally, the anatomic sites of possible exposure should be tested. Testing can be done with cell culture, nucleic acid amplification testing (NAAT), direct immunofluorescence, EIA, and nucleic acid hybridization testing.

> ⚑ **CAUTION!**
>
> The erythromycin 0.05% ointment given as prophylaxis at the time of birth does not prevent opthalmia neonatorum caused by *C. trachomatis*, and topical therapy is insufficient for treatment.

> ⚹ **TIPS & TRICKS**
>
> There is good evidence to support the use of urine samples or self-collected vaginal swabs for NAAT testing for chlamydia infections. This has the benefit of avoiding potentially unnecessary pelvic examinations.

Treatment

Treating pregnant women is important to prevent the spread of disease among sexual partners and transmission to the fetus during childbirth. Coinfection with other STIs should be considered and treated appropriately. Sexual partners should be treated.

Recommended regimens of treatment during pregnancy include:

Azithromycin 1 g po in one dose

or

Amoxicillin 500 mg po tid × 7 days

or

Erythromycin base 500 mg qid × 7 days

or

Erythromycin base 250 mg qid × 14 days

or

Erythromycin ethylsuccinate 800 mg qid × 7 days

or

Erythromycin ethylsuccinate 400 mg qid × 14 days

Erythromycin use is accompanied by gastrointestinal symptoms and its efficacy is compromised because of poor adherence. All three agents, when used properly, have equal efficacy in pregnancy and the same impact on pregnancy outcomes. Test of cure is recommended 3 to 4 weeks following the treatment of pregnant women. Because reinfection rates are high, repeat testing 3 to 6 months after initial infection is also recommended.

> ⚹ **TIPS & TRICKS**
>
> Directly observed administration of a single dose of azithromycin is safe and effective in pregnancy and may improve cure rates because of increased adherence to the treatment regimen.

Gonorrhea

Clinical characteristics

Gonorrhea is caused by the Gram-negative diplococcus *Neisseria gonorrheae* usually affecting the columnar epithelium of mucosal surfaces. Infection rates in pregnancy range from 1% up to 7.8% depending on geographic region and population characteristics.

Up to 50% of gonorrhea genital tract infections in women are asymptomatic, as are most rectal and pharyngeal infections. If a woman presents with symptoms, these include vaginal discharge and dysuria. Examination of the cervix shows mucopurulent discharge, hyperemia, and contact bleeding, consistent with the diagnosis of cervicitis. Up to 3% of infected patients may go on to develop disseminated gonococcal infection (DGI).

Maternal and fetal effects

Gonorrhea during pregnancy can result in preterm premature rupture of membranes, preterm labor, chorioamnionitis, and postpartum endometritis. Diagnosis of gonorrhea in the first trimester is associated with a higher rate of preterm birth later in the pregnancy.

Infection in the neonate is usually due to exposure to cervical exudate during birth, but can also occur as a result of exposure from prolonged rupture of membranes. Gonococcal ophthalmia neonatorum is one of the more severe manifestations of neonatal gonorrhea infection, and can lead to blindness and perforation of the globe of the eye. Rates of infection have decreased dramatically with universal neonatal administration of prophylactic erythromycin 0.5% ointment. DGI may occur in neonates, and can result in sepsis, meningitis, and arthritis.

Diagnosis

Gonorrhea is most commonly diagnosed by cultures of secretions. The sensitivity is high for genital samples and repeat testing should be performed if symptoms persist despite treatment. Nucleic acid amplification tests offer good sensitivity (greater than 90%) for vaginal and endocervical sampling, but the positive predictive value is low in some populations with a low prevalence of disease. These tests are not available commercially for rectal and pharyngeal samples. Culture is preferred over NAATs when antibiotic sensitivity testing is desired.

Treatment

Gonorrohea has historically been treated with penicillin, but with resistance reported in some jurisdictions to be as high as 15%, this treatment is less of an option. Nor are ciprofloxacin and other fluoroquinolones recommended for treatment as resistance to these treatments is rising in Europe and North America. Resistance to azithromycin is also increasing and was found to be as high as 7% in Europe. As of 2008, no resistance was found to spectinomycin or ceftriaxone. While one study demonstrated equivalence in efficacy of ceftriaxone and cefixime, treatment failures with cefixime have also been described.

For treatment of cervicitis secondary to gonorrhea, current recommendations suggest the use of the following:

Cefixime 400 mg po

or

Ceftriaxone 250 mg IM

or

Spectinomycin 2 g IM

In the USA, where spectinomycin is not available, azithromycin 2 g po is a possible treatment regimen.

The above options are all recommended in pregnancy and for the treatment of breast-feeding women with cervicitis. Pharyngeal infection should be treated with ceftriaxone 250 mg IM. If azithromycin and ciprofloxacin resistance have been excluded, azithromycin 2g po or ciprofloxacin 500 mg as single doses may be used.

In some jurisdictions, test of cure among pregnant women is universally recommended. In other areas, test of cure is thought to be necessary only in cases of persistent symptoms, suspicion of antimicrobial resistance, pharyngeal infection, or possible re-exposure to infection. Follow-up assessment and discussion about compliance and resolution of symptoms is always recommended.

Sexual intercourse should be avoided until women who have been diagnosed with gonorrhea, and their partners, are asymptomatic and have completed a course of treatment. Concurrent treatment for chlamydia should be administered unless chlamydia infection has been excluded with a highly sensitive testing modality (i.e. NAAT).

Ophthalmia neonatorum should be treated parenterally with ceftriaxone 25–50 mg/kg IV or IM up to a maximum of 125 mg. Topical treatment is insufficient and not necessary in this setting.

Herpes simplex virus

Clinical characteristics

Herpes simplex virus (HSV) causes a chronic infection that manifests as intermittent, acute, symptomatic episodes. Because of its chronic nature, HSV is common in the general population. Studies estimate a prevalence of 20% in the general population and a range of 25–65% among pregnant women.

Genital herpes is transmitted sexually, most often during periods of subclinical reactivation or from asymptomatic individuals. The primary episode is generally the most severe. Presentation with a painful genital ulcer, often preceded by symptoms of pain and tingling, is typical. Twenty percent of symptomatic primary infections present with urethritis, cervicitis, and aseptic meningitis. Up to 60% of initial infections, however, are asymptomatic. Infections therefore often go undetected until a nonprimary first episode occurs. Nonprimary first episodes are less symptomatic than primary episodes and are associated with fewer lesions. Recurrences are also much less symptomatic than primary episodes and are associated with shorter durations of viral shedding.

The most severe consequence of maternal herpes infection is transmission to the neonate, usually occurring during the intrapartum period. The neonatal risks are greatest with maternal primary infections, which are thought to occur in 2% of pregnancies. The likelihood of transmission depends on the timing and type of episodes, the presence of maternal antibodies, and the length of exposure to the maternal infection.

SCIENCE REVISITED

Genital herpes can by caused by the HSV type 1 or type 2 viruses. The prevalence of type 2 infections is decreasing, while the prevalence of type 1 infections is increasing. HSV type 1 was traditionally responsible for oral infections, but is now responsible for up to 80% of new genital herpes cases. Still, most cases of neonatal herpes are due to HSV-2.

Maternal and fetal effects

The greatest transmission of HSV from the mother to the neonate occurs with exposure in the genital tract during labor, but transplacental and postnatal infections are possible, and neonatal herpes cases have been reported in women undergoing Cesarean sections with no labor.

The greatest risk of intrapartum transmission to the fetus is during a primary episode of herpes when the virus is acquired close to term and maternal seroconversion has not occurred. In this setting there is an approximate 50% chance of transmission to the fetus. Many of these primary episodes are asymptomatic, which explains why 50–80% of neonatal herpes cases occur in women with no known clinical history of herpes.

Neonatal herpes is rare, but causes significant morbidity and mortality. Incidence rates in the USA and Canada range from 5.9 to 60 per 100,000 live births. In the UK rates are reported as low as 1 in 60,000 live births. Infections can be localized to the skin, eyes, and mouth, may involve the central nervous system, or may present as disseminated disease.

SCIENCE REVISITED

Neonates with disease isolated in the skin, eyes, and mouth have the best prognosis with a less than 2% chance of long-term morbidity with treatment and a very rare incidence of death. Central nervous system disease presents with encephalitis and has a 70% chance of causing long-term neurologic morbidity. Disseminated disease has the worst prognosis with a 17% risk of long-term morbidity and a 30% risk of death.

Primary infection during pregnancy can cause antenatal fetal exposure to the virus and result, very rarely, in congenital herpes. This is characterized by chorioretinitis, hydrocephalus, and microcephaly. Antenatal infection may also be responsible for adverse pregnancy outcomes such as preterm birth, preterm premature rupture of membranes, fetal growth restriction, and intrauterine fetal demise.

Diagnosis and screening

Screening is not recommended in asymptomatic women. Serologic testing may be recommended in women whose partners have a history of HSV to counsel for prevention of HSV acquisition in pregnancy.

The diagnosis of HSV involves assessment of clinical characteristics, culture or PCR of genital lesions, and occasionally type-specific antibody testing. Culture from samples obtained from vesicles is 94% sensitive while those from ulcers are 70% sensitive. A Tzanck smear, showing giant nucleated cells, can be used for diagnosis, but is not as reliable as laboratory testing. PCR assays are much more sensitive and specific than viral culture.

Treatment

The goal of management of herpes during pregnancy is to reduce the risk of neonatal herpes while optimizing the care of the mother. Treatment algorithms differ depending on the type of herpes episode and how the infection manifests.

For a primary episode in pregnancy, acyclovir treatment should be administered to reduce the duration and severity of the symptoms. Because viral shedding is thought to be highest after a primary infection and may continue for several weeks after the resolution of symptoms, Caesarean delivery is recommended for any primary infection identified in the third trimester.

When a first episode is identified, type-specific viral culture (and/or PCR where available) should be undertaken, and HSV antibody testing can be performed. If the mother is found to have antibodies against the type of HSV isolated, this probably represents a nonprimary first episode or a recurrence, and the likelihood of effects on the fetus is reduced.

The management of recurrences is debated. Canadian and US guidelines recommend Caesarean delivery for any herpes lesion at the time of labor, while UK guidelines suggest that if the lesion is the result of a recurrence of infection, Caesarean is not always necessary. Transmission of infection to the fetus often occurs in women without any lesions because of asymptomatic shedding of the virus. Several randomized placebo-controlled trials and meta-analyses have been performed looking at the impact of acyclovir and valacylcovir prophylaxis starting at 36 weeks gestation. These studies have shown a decrease in viral shedding as a result of treatment. They have also shown a reduction in the number of lesions and a decreased need for Caesarean delivery at term.

★ TIPS & TRICKS

Antiviral prophylaxis after 36 weeks gestation is recommended in women with a history of HSV to prevent transmission through asymptomatic shedding as well as to reduce the number of Caesarean sections performed because of recurrence close to term.

Doses of antiviral drugs are:

Primary infection:

o Acyclovir 200 mg five times daily for 5–10 days

Recurrence:

o Acyclovir 200 mg five times daily for 5 days

Prophylaxis – history of HSV infection:

o Acyclovir 400 mg three times daily from 36 weeks until delivery
o Valacylclovir 500 mg twice daily from 36 weeks until delivery

Studies have not shown any increase in congenital anomalies or adverse pregnancy outcomes with acyclovir exposure.

Human papilloma virus

Clinical characteristics

Human papilloma virus (HPV) is common, with many subtypes causing infections of the anogenital epithelium. While most infections are asymptomatic or subclinical, high-risk subtypes can lead to precancerous lesions and low-risk subtypes can cause genital warts and recurrent respiratory papillomatosis. Fifty to seventy percent of sexually active individuals will be infected at some point in their lives, but because of changing demographics and differences in clearance of the virus, prevalence varies widely. Rates of HPV prevalence among young women are high.

Canadian studies show a range of prevalence among young women from 29% up to 73% in certain settings, and some studies have shown prevalence rates as high as 90%.

HPV is transmitted sexually through skin-to-skin contact and, as such, condom use confers only 60% protection against infection. The number of lifetime sexual partners is the strongest risk factor for HPV infection. Other risk factors include smoking and exposure to tobacco smoke, immunosuppression, high number of pregnancies, other sexually transmitted infections, inadequate diet, and genetic susceptibility.

Most infections are asymptomatic and subclinical. The low-risk subtypes may cause genital warts, which are flat or pedunculated growths found on the genital mucosa. Warts are usually asymptomatic, but may cause pain or pruritus and may also bleed or cause local discharge. The low-risk subtypes are also responsible for recurrent respiratory papillomatosis, a condition thought to affect neonates and infants secondary to mother-to-child transmission of the virus.

SCIENCE REVISITED

Vaccines are available to prevent the transmission of HPV and are the most reliable form of prevention available. A cohort of women who became pregnant shortly after the administration of the quadrivalent HPV vaccine was studied. There was no observed difference in the rates of adverse pregnancy outcomes, fetal loss, or congenital anomalies among recently vaccinated women and those women who received placebo. Among women who received the vaccine during pregnancy, no increased risks of spontaneous abortion or congenital anomalies were noted. Despite the lack of evidence showing any fetal risk with vaccine exposure, administration during pregnancy is not recommended.

Maternal and fetal effects

HPV infection has not been shown to be associated with any adverse pregnancy outcomes.

Genital warts may increase in size or number during pregnancy, and may become more susceptible to bleeding and more difficult to treat.

Conflicting evidence exists regarding the possibility of mother-to-child transmission of HPV, the mode of transmission, and of the implications of this possible transmission. While HPV is known to cross the placenta, a large case-control study showed no association between genital warts and congenital anomalies.

Mother-to-child-transmission of HPV types 6 and 11 may cause neonatal recurrent respiratory papillomatosis. DNA from these HPV subtypes has been isolated from genital warts and papillomas in the respiratory tract, and the single best predictor of juvenile recurrent respiratory papillomatosis is the presence of maternal genital warts during pregnancy. Still, recurrent respiratory papillomatosis is extremely rare and the risk does not decrease with Caesarean delivery. Caesarean is only recommended if the warts result in a pelvic outlet obstruction or if the already friable warts bleed excessively during the vaginal birth.

Diagnosis and screening

Universal testing for HPV is not recommended. If warts are present, their diagnosis is based on clinical features. If they are at all abnormal in appearance, pigmented, persistent, or refractory to treatment, biopsy may be indicated.

Treatment

Genital warts in pregnancy may not respond readily to treatment and regression generally occurs in the postpartum period. Many of the usual treatment methods for the genital warts are contraindicated in pregnancy, but if treatment is undertaken due to patient request or because the symptoms are disruptive, options are as follows:

- Trichloroacetic acid (85%) directly applied to lesions
- Cryotherapy of lesions
- Carbon dioxide laser
- Surgical removal

Imiquimod, podophyllin, 5-fluorouracil, and interferon are not recommended in pregnancy.

Cervical cytology changes caused by HPV should be referred to colposcopy appropriately.

Biopsies are acceptable, but endocervical curet-tage is contraindicated in pregnancy. Unless invasive cervical cancer is suspected or confirmed, treatment with cervical conization for precancerous lesions is not indicated in pregnancy.

✋ CAUTION!

Endocervical curettage is contraindicated in pregnancy. Cervical conization should be reserved for cases where invasive cervical cancer is suspected. Such cases are best managed by a gynecologic-oncology specialist.

Syphilis

Clinical characteristics

Syphilis is a systemic illness caused by the spirochete *Treponema pallidum*. It is transmitted sexually or by vertical transmission at any stage of pregnancy. World wide, the incidence of syphilis is increasing. Prevalence among pregnant women ranges from 1% to 17.5% in some regions. Globally, rates of congenital syphilis have increased 23% from 8.2 cases per 100,000 live births in 2005 to 10.1 cases per 100,000 live births in 2008.

⚗ SCIENCE REVISITED

Data from WHO lead to estimates that in a year, one million pregnancies are affected by syphilis, with 460,000 of these ending in stillbirth or abortion, 270,000 pregnancies complicated by prematurity and low birthweight, and 270,000 babies born with congenital syphilis world wide.

Syphilis initially presents with lesions, known as chancres, at the site of infection; in the urogenital region, the mouth, or the rectum. Progression is divided into clinical stages, all of which may be seen during pregnancy:

- Primary syphilis: chancre at the infection site
- Secondary syphilis: involvement of skin, mucocutaneous tissue, lymphadenopathy

- Latent syphilis: serologic evidence of disease without clinical manifestations
- Tertiary syphilis:
  o Cardiac and gummatous lesions
  o Neurosyphilis: altered mental status, loss of vibration sense, altered auditory and ophthalmic sensation, stroke, meningitis, cranial nerve dysfunction

Maternal and fetal effects

Transmission of syphilis to the fetus and newborn, and the consequent adverse pregnancy and neonatal outcomes, decreases dramatically with treatment during pregnancy. Because of this, universal screening at the beginning of pregnancy is necessary. Many recommendations call for a second point of screening later in pregnancy, especially in high prevalence settings or among high-risk individuals.

Syphilis during pregnancy, especially when left untreated, can lead to stillbirths, neonatal death, and congenital syphilis in the newborn. Among women with primary syphilis that is untreated, transmission to the fetus occurs in 70–100% of cases, while among those with early latent syphilis, transmission occurs in 40% of cases. Among women who are treated for syphilis in pregnancy, transmission to the fetus drops to 1–2%.

Congenital syphilis is defined as an illness where *Treponema pallidum* can be identified in lesional samples, placental samples, the umbilical cord, or in autopsy specimens. Infants are thought to have congenital syphilis if they have a positive treponemal test and either physical examiation evidence of congenital syphilis, radiographic evidence of congenital syphilis, positive CSF VDRL test, elevated CSF cell count or protein, or positive IgM by antibody testing or enzyme-linked immunosorbent assay. Ultrasound findings include fetal hepatomegaly, ascites, and hydrops. These findings indicate a more severe infection and one that may be refractory to treatment.

Early congenital syphilis presents in the first 2 years of life, while late congenital syphilis presents at any time in the individual's lifespan. Neonates affected by congenital syphilis are initially asymptomatic, and early congenital syphilis usually presents 3 to 8 months postnatally. Clinical findings include a blistering skin rash, hepatomegaly, splenomegaly, jaundice, respiratory distress, pseudoparalysis, fever, or bleeding. Bone changes can be seen on X-ray. Serologic testing should be performed on all infants at risk because up to 60% of those affected will be asymptomatic.

Diagnosis and screening

Most jurisdictions consider the universal screening of all pregnant women to be the standard of care. The WHO has deemed universal screening to be cost-effective and of proven benefit.

🜂 SCIENCE REVISITED

Screening is recommended at every woman's first prenatal visit. Subsequent testing is recommended in the third trimester, either universally, or for women at high risk of contracting syphilis during their pregnancy. This group includes women living in geographic regions of high syphilis prevalence, adolescents, women with other STIs, those living in poverty, and those involved in the sex trade or in illicit drug use.

Darkfield microscopy of specimens from affected tissue is the standard diagnostic test for *T. pallidum* infection, but is not commercially available. Serologic diagnosis is made with non-treponemal and treponemal testing. Both tests are required for accurate diagnosis and monitoring of disease activity. Screening and testing strategies differ between jurisdictions.

Treponemal testing is done with various immunoassays, such as fluorescent treponemal antibody absorbed tests (FTA-ABS), *T. pallidum* passive particle agglutination assay (TP-PA), and other enzyme immunoassays. Once positive, only 15–25% of affected individuals become serologically negative despite treatment, so the test cannot be used to detect the response to treatment.

Nontreponemal tests include the VDRL (Venereal Diseases Research Laboratory) and RPR (rapid plasma regain) tests. Because of the desire for a high sensitivity, these are often associated with a high false-positive rate in women with autoimmune disease or a history of injection drug use, hepatitis, Epstein–Barr viral infections, and in women who are older. Once positive results are confirmed by using treponemal specific tests, the titers obtained with the VDRL or RPR tests correlate with disease activity. The titers decrease with treatment and can be used to monitor disease activity. As the results of VDRL and RPR tests are not interchangeable, disease monitoring should be performed with only one of the two types of test used sequentially on the same patient.

Treatment

Treatment of pregnant women with syphilis significantly reduces the rate of congenital syphilis. *T. pallidum* can reside in anatomical areas not accessible to all forms of penicillin and, as such, penicillin G, or benzathine penicillin, is considered the only adequate form of treatment in pregnancy. Those women reporting penicillin allergies should be desensitized and then given benzathine penicillin.

Dosing is as follows:

- Primary and secondary syphilis: Benzathine penicillin 2.4 million units IM × 1
- Early latent syphilis: Benzathine penicillin 2.4 million units IM × 1
- Late latent or tertiary syphilis: Benzathine penicillin 2.4 million units IM × 3 in one week intervals
- Congenital syphilis in an infant: Benzathine penicillin 50,000 units/kg IM, to a maximum of 2.4 million units IM × 1

★ TIPS & TRICKS

In some jurisdictions, benzathine penicillin is not available in pharmacies and can only be obtained from local departments of public health.

Following treatment, clinical status and serology should be reviewed monthly until delivery, especially in women at high-risk for reinfection. If syphilis is diagnosed after 20 weeks gestation, detailed ultrasounds should be performed to assess for expected response to treatment.

Table 15.1. Characteristics of common vaginitides

	Vulvovaginal candidiasis	Bacterial vaginosis	Trichomoniasis
Symptoms	Pruritus, vulvar erythema	Malodor, occasional pruritus	Vulvar irritation, dyspareunia
Discharge	Thick-white, curd-like	Thick, adherent	Thick, purulent, green, frothy
Vaginal pH	<4.5	>4.5	>4.5
Wet mount saline microscopy	Pseudohyphae	Clue cells	Motile trichomonads
Whiff tTest	Negative	Positive, "fishy" odor	Often positive

Partners should be treated, and the newborn should be evaluated at regular intervals in the postnatal period.

Vaginitides

Vaginitides are common among pregnant women and may be associated with adverse pregnancy outcomes. Vaginal discharge in these cases must be differentiated from the physiologic discharge commonly experienced by most pregnant women. Presentation and diagnosis of common vaginitides is summarized in Table 15.1.

Bacterial vaginosis

Clinical characteristics

Bacterial vaginosis is a polymicrobial condition characterized by alteration in the balance of normal vaginal flora. The hydrogen-peroxide producing *Lactobacillus* species, which usually comprise 95% of vaginal flora, are replaced by higher concentrations of pathologic species, such as *Gardnerella vaginalis*, *Mycoplasma*, *Ureaplasma*, and other anaerobic bacteria. Vaginal discharge and odor develop, and the condition has been linked with several pregnancy and postpartum complications.

Bacterial vaginosis is very common and prevalence ranges among groups based on age, race, education, and socioeconomic status. Survey data from the United States shows an overall prevalence of 29%, while prevalence in pregnancy has been estimated between 10 and 30%, with a Canadian study showing a rate of 16.7% in the first trimester and 12% at the time of labor.

Other risk factors include smoking, early sexual debut, new sexual partner, lack of condom use, vaginal douching, and race or ethnicity. In pregnancy, the prevalence of bacterial vaginosis has been shown to be higher in women of low socioeconomic status, ethnic minority groups in the United States, and those with a history of a previous low birth weight infant. Recent analyses have implicated vitamin D deficiency in pregnant women as a risk factor, which may contribute in part to the ethnic differences found in the prevalence of bacterial vaginosis. It remains unclear what mechanisms lead to the development of the imbalance characterizing bacterial vaginosis and as to whether a sexually acquired pathogen plays any role.

Maternal and fetal effects

Bacterial vaginosis can cause symptoms of discharge, odor, and pruritus.

Evidence exists for the association of bacterial vaginosis with an increased risk of late miscarriage, preterm labor, preterm premature rupture of membranes, and preterm birth. Maternal complications include chorioamnionitis and postpartum endometritis.

☙ SCIENCE REVISITED

The link between bacterial vagniosis and adverse pregnancy outcomes is tenuous. While the rates of bacterial vaginosis in women who give birth prematurely have been shown to be double the rates among those who give birth at term, only 10–30% of women who are BV positive go on to deliver prematurely. The alteration of flora may trigger the mucosal immune system through the release of several inflammatory cytokines and prostaglandins. Women display varying host immune responses to this release and so the rates of symptomatic infections and adverse obstetric outcomes vary. The pro-inflammatory cytokines are thought to lead to the development of preterm birth and preterm premature rupture of membranes.

Diagnosis and screening

A diagnosis of bacterial vaginosis can be made clinically, microbiologically with a Gram stain, or molecularly with PCR. Clinical diagnosis is based on the presence of three out of four of Amsel's criteria:

- The presence of a homogeneous, low-viscosity, milk-like discharge.
- A vaginal pH of greater than 4.5.
- The release of an amine, fish-like odor upon addition of 10% potassium hydroxide solution to a drop of vaginal discharge.
- The presence of clue cells on saline wet mount. The clue cells are epithelial cells with a stippled, granular appearance, and obscured borders secondary to attached organisms.

A microbiological diagnosis is made by Gram stain of the vaginal discharge. Quantification of the *Lactobacillus* morphotypes compared to the pathogenic bacteria yields a score, like the commonly used Nugent score, to identify the presence of bacterial vaginosis.

☆ TIPS & TRICKS

Testing for bacterial vaginosis should only be conducted on symptomatic women. Asymptomatic women with a history of preterm birth may be screened in pregnancy to attempt to decrease the risk of recurrent preterm birth.

Screening in pregnancy remains a debated issue. Many studies have shown conflicting results regarding the benefits of screening to prevent preterm birth. If a woman presents with a persistent discharge, screening and treatment of a positive result is warranted to provide relief from symptoms.

In women with a history of preterm birth or preterm premature rupture of membranes, routine screening at 12–16 weeks and according treatment may reduce the risk of recurrence of the adverse outcome, although this has not been consistently proven.

Treatment

Treatment in pregnancy is widely debated in the literature. Up to 50% of cases resolve spontaneously throughout pregnancy, while in other cases, regardless of treatment, infections tend to recur. Certainly, treatment is recommended for the relief of symptoms. Many studies with oral preparations show cure rates from 70% to 92.5% at 2–4 weeks following treatment.

The impact of treatment of BV infection on rates of adverse pregnancy outcomes is not clear. The treatment of women with a low risk for preterm birth does not reduce the rates of preterm birth, low birth weight, or preterm premature rupture of membranes. For women at high risk of adverse pregnancy outcomes, numerous large trials, systematic reviews and meta-analyses have shown a reduction in the risk of preterm birth, preterm premature rupture of membranes, and low birth weight infants with oral treatment early in pregnancy.

Treatment regimens:

- Preferred: Metronidazole 500 mg po bid × 7 days
- Alternatives: Metronidazole 250 mg po tid × 7 days *or* clindamycin 300 mg po bid × 7 days.

While oral agents have been shown to reduce the risk of adverse pregnancy outcomes, vaginal agents have not had these effects. Because there is a risk of a subclinical upper genital tract infection, it makes sense that systemic therapy would be more efficacious than local therapy. Vaginal clindamycin cream, especially when given later in pregnancy, has been shown to increase the risk of neonatal infections and is not recommended. Oral metronidazole has not been shown to have teratogenic or mutagenic effects on the fetus in many studies, but in a few studies its use has been associated with higher rates of preterm birth.

Because of high recurrence rates, rescreening and retreatment can be considered in pregnancy for women at high risk of adverse outcomes. The probability of recurrence is unaffected by treatment of sexual partners and routine treatment of partners is not recommended.

Vulvovaginal candidiasis

Clinical characteristics

Vulvovaginal candidiasis is a common fungal infection, with 75% of women experiencing at least one infection in their lifetime. Ninety percent of cases are caused by *Candida albicans*, while the other 10% are caused by other *Candida* species or by *Saccharomyces cerevisiae*. In pregnancy, the prevalence has been found to be 12.5% in a population of asymptomatic women. Because pregnancy results in increased levels of circulating estrogens and the deposition of glycogen vaginally, pregnant women have a twofold increased risk of vulvovaginal candidiasis.

Candida albicans is a commensal agent in the normal vagina. With an overgrowth of *Candida* (and other not completely delineated mechanisms), an inflammatory reaction is induced, producing the following symptoms: vulvar pruritus, pain, erythema, and swelling. Dyspareunia and external dysuria are also common symptoms. A thick curd-like discharge is a distinguishing feature of the condition.

Maternal and fetal effects

Studies assessing the impact of *Candida* infection on the rates of preterm birth have had mixed results. A study looking at infectious predictors of preterm birth found no association between the detection of *Candida* infection in the first trimester and preterm birth or low birth weight infants.

Rare cases of intrauterine transmission of *Candida* to the fetus have been described. Red, cutaneous lesions on the neonate and white lesions on the placenta are found in these cases of congenital candidiasis. The skin lesions appear in the first week of life and may progress to desquamation or may resolve in 2 to 3 weeks. This is accompanied by a leukemoid reaction in blood counts, and *Candida* can be cultured from the lesions or from the placenta.

Diagnosis

Clinical diagnosis of *Candida* infection can be made in the presence of vulvar pain, pruritus, dysuria, and thick white discharge. A saline wet mount and Gram stain may show yeast, hyphae, or pseudohyphae. Hyphae may be better visualized with a 10% KOH wet mount. Vaginal pH will be normal (<4.5). In a woman with two or more symptoms and a negative wet mount, a vaginal culture may be useful. This is especially the case in recurrent vulvovaginitis to rule out non-*albicans* species of *Candida*. It is important not to screen asymptomatic women since 10–20% of the population may be colonized at any one time with *Candida* and do not warrant treatment.

Treatment

Treatment during pregnancy is directed at relief of symptoms, since eradication is difficult to achieve. The following topical, intravaginal formulations are recommended in pregnancy:

- Butoconazole 2% cream 5 g × 1
- Clotrimazole 1% cream 5 g OD × 7–14 days, *or* 100 mg vaginal tablet OD × 7 days *or* 100 mg vaginal tablet bid × 3 days *or* 500 mg vaginal tablet once
- Miconazole 2% cream 5 g OD × 7 days *or* 100 mg vaginal suppository OD × 7 days *or* 200 mg vaginal suppository OD × 3 days
- Nystatin 100,000 unity vaginal tablet OX × 14 days
- Terconazole 0.4% cream 5 g OD × 7 days *or* 0.8% cream 5 g OD × 3 days *or* 80 mg vaginal suppository OD × 3 days

Treatment with oral fluconazole should be reserved for refractory cases.

SCIENCE REVISITED

Oral fluconazole treatment using doses of 400 mg has been implicated in teratogenesis in animal studies. The usual dose for treatment of vaginal canadiasis is 150 mg. No fetal complications have been identified with treatment in humans using this lower dose.

Trichomonas vaginalis

Clinical characteristics

Trichomonas vaginalis is a motile protozoan and is responsible for one of the most common STIs world wide. Annually, 174 million new cases are identified. Eight million of these new cases are found in North America, 32 million in sub-Saharan Africa, and 74.5 million are found annually in South and Southeast Asia. In pregnancy, prevalence ranges from as low as 2.1% to as high as 27.5%, depending on geographic and patient characteristics.

Prevalence is generally high in resource-poor settings. In the United States, risk factors for *T. vaginalis* include being part of an ethnic minority group, low condom use, multiple sex partners, sex workers, high rates of douching, drug use, and lack of access to healthcare.

Thirty to fifty percent of infections in women are asymptomatic. When symptoms are present, a frothy malodorous yellow-green discharge and vulvar irritation are described. Common complaints include dysuria and dyspareunia. Systemic symptoms are not seen.

Maternal and fetal effects

Trichomonas infection in pregnancy is thought to create a local and systemic inflammatory reaction associated with several adverse pregnancy outcomes including preterm premature rupture of membranes, preterm labor, and low birth weight. A large cohort study controlling for several confounders and assessing women found to be positive on vaginal culture, showed a 40% increase in the rates of preterm births among women infected with *T. vaginalis*. Possible mechanisms for how the *T. vaginalis* parasite my cause preterm birth include its adherence to vaginal walls, its acting as a covector for another parasite, or it creating a direct inflammatory reaction on the cervix and in the uterine decidua. While systemic symptoms are generally not seen, a study looking at the systemic inflammatory response in pregnant women with *Trichomonas* infection showed an increase in the levels of CRP, which may play a role in inducing labor, either at term or at preterm.

Diagnosis and screening

Trichomoniasis can be detected by microscopy or by culture of vaginal secretions. Microscopy of a wet mount of vaginal secretions shows motile flagellated protozoa and yields a varying sensitivity of 38–82%. Its utility lies in the fact that it may provide a point-of-care diagnosis. When trichomoniasis is suspected clinically, and microscopy yields negative results, vaginal secretions should be sent for culture.

Screening is not recommended for all pregnant women because treatment has not been shown to reduce adverse pregnancy outcomes, and some studies have shown an association between treatment and preterm birth.

★ TIPS & TRICKS

Culture using Diamond's medium is much more sensitive and specific compared with culture collected using routine charcoal swabs.

Treatment

The role of treatment is to alleviate symptoms and prevent reinfection. Studies have failed to show that the treatment of trichomoniasis in pregnancy reduces the rate of preterm birth. Treatment may indeed increase rates of preterm birth, and should only be reserved for symptomatic women and their partners.

Metronidazole 2 g orally in a single dose or 500 mg twice daily for 7 days are both safe regimens and are recommended in pregnancy. Vaginal treatment with metronidazole gel is less than 50% as effective as oral treatment and should not be used for this pathogen. Treatment of sexual partners and abstinence during treatment are both necessary for the prevention of reinfection. Test-of-cure is not necessary and retesting should be reserved for women with a persistence of symptoms.

Bibliography

Amsel R, Totten PA, Spiegel CA, et al. Nonspecific vaginitis. Diagnostic criteria and microbial and epidemiologic associations. *Am J Med* 1983 Jan; **74**(1): 14–22.

Aoki F. Genital herpes simplex virus (HSV) infections. In: *Canadian Guidelines on Sexually Transmitted Infections*, 2006 edn, updated January 2008 (Wong T, ed.). Public Health Agency of Canada: Ottawa; 2008.

Banhidy F, Acs N, Puho EH, Czeizel AE. Birth outcomes among pregnant women with genital warts. *Int J Gynecol Obstet* 2010 Feb; **108**(2): 153–154.

Bignell C. *2009* European (IUSTI/WHO) guideline on the diagnosis and treatment of gonorrhoea in adults. *Intern J STD AIDS* 2009 Jul; **20**(7): 453–457.

CDC. Sexually Transmitted Diseases Guidelines, 2010. *MMWR*, 2010 Dec; **59**(RR–12): 1–109.

Cook RL, Hutchison SL, Ostergaard L, et al. Systematic review: noninvasive testing for Chlamydia trachomatis and Neisseria gonorrhoeae. *Ann Intern Med* 2005 Jun; **142**(11): 914–925.

Corey L, Wald A. Maternal and neonatal herpes simplex virus infections. *New Engl J Med* 2009 Oct; **361**(14): 1376–1385.

Cotch MF, Pastorek JG, 2nd, Nugent RP, Hillier SL, Gibbs RS, Martin DH, et al. Trichomonas vaginalis associated with low birth weight and preterm delivery. The Vaginal Infections and Prematurity Study Group. *Sex Transm Dis* 1997 Jul; **24**(6): 353–360.

Doroshenko A, Sherrard J, Pollard AJ. Syphilis in pregnancy and the neonatal period. *Intern J STD AIDS* 2006 Apr; **17**(4): 221–227; quiz 8.

Gardella C, Brown Z. Prevention of neonatal herpes. *BJOG (Intern J Obstet Gynecol)*. 2011 Jan; **118**(2): 187–192.

Genc M, Ledger WJ. Syphilis in pregnancy. *Sex Transm Infect* 2000 Apr; **76**(2): 73–79.

Lanjouw E, Ossewaarde JM, Stary A, et al. 2010 European guideline for the management of Chlamydia trachomatis infections. *Intern J STD AIDS* 2010 Nov; **21**(11): 729–737.

Meyers DS, Halvorson H, Luckhaupt S. Screening for chlamydial infection: an evidence update for the U.S. Preventive Services Task Force. *Ann Intern Med* 2007 Jul; **147**(2): 135–142.

Nygren P, Fu R, Freeman M, et al Evidence on the benefits and harms of screening and treating pregnant women who are asymptomatic for bacterial vaginosis: an update review for the U.S. Preventive Services Task Force. *Ann Intern Med* 2008 Feb; **148**(3): 220–233.

Soong D, Einarson A. Vaginal yeast infections during pregnancy. *Can Fam Phys* 2009 Mar; **55**(3): 255–256.

Wong T (ed.). *Canadian Guidelines on Sexually Transmitted Infections*, 2006 edn, updated January 2010. Canadian Public Health Agency: Ottawa, 2008.

Yudin MH, Money DM. Screening and management of bacterial vaginosis in pregnancy. *J Obstet Gynecol Can* 2008 Aug; **30**(8): 702–716.

Treatment of Sexually Transmitted Infections in Pregnancy

Silvia T. Linares and Lisa M. Hollier

Department of Obstetrics, Gynecology & Reproductive Sciences, University of Texas Houston Medical School, Houston, TX, USA

Introduction

Sexually transmitted infections during pregnancy affect the mother and can affect the developing fetus or the newborn at delivery. STIs are strongly related to preterm delivery, low birth weight and increased morbidity and mortality. Appropriate screening and prompt treatment are essential to prevent maternal and fetal complications. All pregnant women should be asked about STIs, counseled about the possibility of perinatal infections, and provided appropriate access to treatment, if needed. Their sex partners should also be included whenever possible. Physicians and other healthcare providers play a critical role in preventing and treating STDs. This chapter discusses screening and treatment for the most prevalent STIs among pregnant women.

There are a number of pregnancy-associated factors that need to be considered when planning the appropriate treatment for STIs among pregnant women. Important maternal adaptations take place during pregnancy, including an increase in the plasma volume of about 45–50%. The glomerular filtration rate (GFR), as measured by creatinine clearance, increases by approximately 50% by the end of the first trimester to a peak of around 180 mL/min. Some therapeutic regimens are given at higher doses for pregnant women (e.g. prophylaxis for HSV during the last weeks of pregnancy) than for nonpregnant women. Some widely used medications for the treatment of STIs are not considered safe for use during pregnancy due to potential complications for the newborn (e.g. tetracyclines and fluoroquinolones). In addition, the variable transplacental passage of various antibiotics may have implications for fetal treatment of in-utero infections (e.g. erythromycin may not prevent congenital syphilis due to the variability of transplacental passage of the antibiotic).

Genital herpes

Genital herpes is a chronic, life-long viral infection and is one of the most common sexually transmitted infections world wide. An estimated 50 million people in the United States have been infected, but the vast majority (>80%) have not been diagnosed. Herpes simplex virus type-1 and type-2 both cause genital ulcers and can be transmitted to the fetus or newborn during pregnancy and delivery. While HSV-2 is often thought of as the "genital" pathogen, an increasing number of new genital infections are caused by HSV-1, particularly among young women. Using

Sexually Transmitted Diseases, First Edition. Edited by Richard H. Beigi.
© 2012 John Wiley & Sons, Ltd. Published 2012 by John Wiley & Sons, Ltd.

population-based serologic studies, the prevalence of HSV-2 is higher among women (20.9%) than men (11.5%). In addition, there are striking racial/ethnic disparities with a seroprevalence rates nearly three times higher among non-Hispanic black women (48%).

Approximately 2% of women will become infected with herpes during pregnancy. The risk for transmission to the neonate from an infected mother is 30–60% when the mother acquires HSV near the time of delivery. For women with recurrent genital HSV the risk of transmission with a vaginal delivery is only 3%. Among women with a history of recurrent disease, and no visible lesions at delivery, the transmission risk has been estimated to be 2/10,000.

Because the risk of transmission is highest with new infections in pregnancy, approximately 80% of affected infants are born to women who have no history of clinically evident genital herpes. Mortality for neonatal herpes has decreased significantly; however, 30% of infants with disseminated disease will die and 20% of survivors will have neurologic sequelae.

Diagnosis

Because the clinical appearance of genital ulcers can be misleading, a diagnosis of genital herpes should be confirmed by laboratory testing. For women with genital ulcers or similar lesions, cell culture and polymerase chain reaction (PCR) are the preferred diagnostic tests for herpes simplex virus infection. PCR assays for HSV DNA are more sensitive than cell culture and are becoming more widespread. While they have not been FDA-cleared for testing genital specimens, many individual laboratories have developed their own PCR assays for clinical use. It is important to remember that a negative culture or PCR does not rule out the diagnosis of herpes because of the imperfect sensitivity of the tests. Serologic tests for HSV antibodies are a useful adjunct for confirming diagnosis and can also be used for screening asymptomatic individuals. Because nearly all HSV-2 infections are sexually acquired, the presence of type-specific HSV-2 antibody implies anogenital infection. The presence of HSV-1 antibody alone is more difficult to interpret because of the frequency of oral infections.

While all pregnant women should be asked whether they have a history of genital herpes, routine serologic screening of all pregnant women for HSV-2 antibodies is not currently recommended.

Treatment

Acyclovir, famciclovir, and valacyclovir are all FDA pregnancy category B medications. These drugs are all approved for the treatment of primary genital herpes, the treatment of episodes of recurrent disease, and the daily treatment for suppression of recurrent outbreaks. Data from registries does not suggest an increased risk for major birth defects among women treated with acyclovir during the first trimester. However, data regarding prenatal exposure to valacyclovir and famciclovir is too limited to provide useful information on pregnancy outcomes.

Antiviral treatment may be administered orally to pregnant women with first episode genital herpes or severe recurrent herpes. Examples of regimens are listed in Table 16.1. The oral treatment of primary or first-episode infections can be extended for more than 10 days for patients whose lesions are incompletely healed. Acyclovir should be administered IV to pregnant women with severe HSV infection or in disseminated herpetic infections. A recommended regimen is acyclovir 5–10 mg/kg IV every 8 hours for 2–7 days or until clinical improvement is observed, followed by oral antiviral therapy to complete at least 10 days of total therapy. There are no clinical trials which suggest dosing modifications during pregnancy. Dosing interval modifications are required for individuals with renal impairment.

A recent Cochrane review of the use of third trimester antiviral prophylaxis to prevent the maternal herpes virus recurrences and neonatal infection concluded that there is insufficient evidence to determine if antiviral prophylaxis reduces the incidence of neonatal herpes, but prophylaxis does reduce both viral shedding and recurrences at delivery as well as reducing Cesarean delivery performed for HSV (Table 16.1). The risks, benefits, and alternatives to antenatal prophylaxis should be discussed with women who have a history of herpes, and prophylaxis should be initiated if they desire intervention.

Table 16.1. Antivirals for genital herpes in pregnancy

	Primary or first episode	Recurrent episodes	Suppression
Acyclovir	400 mg orally tid for 7-10 days	400 mg orally tid for 5 days *or* 800 mg orally bid for 5 days *or* 800 mg orally tid for 2 days	400 mg orally tid from 36 weeks until delivery
Valacyclovir	1000 mg orally bid for 7-10 days	500 mg orally bid for 3 days *or* 1000 mg orally daily for 5 days	500 mg orally bid from 36 weeks until delivery
Famciclovir	250 mg orally tid for 7-10 days	125 mg orally bid for 5 days *or* 1000 mg orally bid for 1 day *or* 500 mg orally once then 250 mg orally bid for 2 days	No data

✶ TIPS & TRICKS

A recent Cochrane review of use third trimester antiviral prophylaxis to prevent the maternal herpes virus recurrences and neonatal infection concluded that there insufficient evidence to determine if antiviral prophylaxis reduces the incidence of neonatal herpes; however, prophylaxis does reduce both viral shedding and recurrences at delivery as well as reducing Cesarean delivery performed for HSV.

At the onset of labor, all women should be questioned about signs and symptoms of genital herpes (including prodrome), and all women should be examined for herpetic lesions. Cesarean delivery is recommended for women with active genital herpetic lesions at the onset of labor to reduce the risk of neonatal transmission; however, Cesarean delivery does not completely eliminate the risk for HSV transmission to the infant. Women without symptoms or signs of genital herpes or its prodrome can deliver vaginally.

Syphilis

Antepartum syphilis can profoundly affect pregnancy outcome by causing preterm labor, fetal death, and neonatal infection by either transplacental or perinatal infection. Fortunately, of the many congenital infections, syphilis is the most readily prevented and also the most susceptible to therapy.

Diagnosis

The diagnosis of syphilis is usually made using serologic tests, though, in early syphilis, direct darkfield examination to show the presence of spirochetes in lesion exudate is the definitive method of diagnosis. The CDC continues to recommend that nontreponemal serologic tests (e.g. VDRL and RPR) be used for screening and follow-up; while treponemal tests (e.g. FTA-ABS, TP-PA) be used to confirm the infection. Automatable treponemal enzyme and chemiluminescence immunoassays (EIA/CIA) are being used by certain laboratories in reverse sequence syphilis screening. The use of treponemal tests first identifies both persons with treated and untreated syphilis, thus reducing its predictive value, especially in populations with a low prevalence of syphilis. Pregnant women with reactive treponemal screening tests should have confirmatory testing with nontreponemal tests with titers.

Most states mandate screening at the first prenatal visit for all women; there is variation in the content of the statutes about the number and timing of tests. States with a heavy burden of infectious syphilis in women tend to require more prenatal testing. The CDC advises a retest early in the third trimester (28 weeks) and at delivery, patients at high risk, and those who live in areas with a high prevalence of syphilis, as well as any patient previously untested. Any woman who delivers a stillborn infant after 20 weeks' gestation should be tested for syphilis.

Treatment

Parenteral penicillin G is the drug of choice for the treatment of all stages of syphilis. Penicillin is effective for preventing maternal transmission to the fetus and for treating fetal infection. While evidence to determine the optimal penicillin regimen is limited, pregnant women should receive the penicillin dose appropriate for the stage of syphilis (Table 16.2). Tetracycline and doxycycline generally are not used during pregnancy. Tetracyclines can cause yellow-brown discoloration of the fetal deciduous teeth. Erythromycin and azithromycin should not be used, because neither reliably cures maternal infection nor treats an infected fetus. Data is insufficient to recommend ceftriaxone for the treatment of maternal infection and the prevention of congenital syphilis.

Pregnant women who have a history of a type-I hypersensitivity allergic reaction to penicillin should be desensitized, and subsequently treated with penicillin. Oral stepwise penicillin dose challenge or skin testing might be helpful in identifying women at risk for acute allergic reactions. There are two options for desensitization IV and oral, both are effective but the oral regimen is cheaper, safer, and easier to perform over 4–12 hours. One desensitization regimen is detailed in Table 16.3.

The rate of treatment failure may be increased in pregnant patients with early syphilis, particularly secondary syphilis (2–5%), and therefore some experts recommend a second injection of benzathine penicillin G, 2.4 million units IM one week after the first injection. Because the risk of treatment failure is congenital syphilis, missed doses are not acceptable for pregnant patients undergoing treatment for late latent syphilis. Pregnant women who miss any doses should repeat the entire course of therapy.

When syphilis is diagnosed during the second half of pregnancy, management should include a sonographic fetal evaluation for congenital syphilis, but this evaluation should not delay therapy.

Within hours after treatment, patients can develop an acute complication termed the Jarisch–Herxheimer reaction. Although the reaction occurs in 10–25% of patients overall, the reaction is much more common in primary and secondary syphilis. Symptoms include fever, chills, myalgias, and headache. Contractions, fetal heart rate decelerations, decreased fetal movement, fetal distress, and fetal death can occur with treatment in pregnancy. Hospitalization may be warranted in some cases for maternal and fetal monitoring. Symptoms last for 12–24 hours and are usually self-limiting. Patients can be treated symptomatically with antipyretics.

The CDC recommends that the response to therapy be monitored with clinical and serologic examination at 28–32 weeks and at delivery. Because of the morbidity of congenital syphilis, more frequent testing such as every 3 months may be appropriate.

Gonorrhea

Gonorrhea is the second most commonly reported notifiable disease in the United States though rates of gonorrhea have declined significantly over the last 30 years. Rates of infection among women still exceed rates among men (105.5 cases vs. 91.9 per 100,000 population

Table 16.2. Recommended regimen for syphilis during pregnancy from Centers for Disease Control

Primary, secondary, or early latent stage	Benzathine penicillin G, 2.4 million units IM in a single dose
Late latent stage or syphilis of unknown duration	Benzathine penicillin G, 2.4 million units IM once a week for 3 consecutive weeks
Neurosyphilis	Aqueous crystalline penicillin G, 3–4 million units IV every 4 hours or 18–24 million units daily as continuous infusion, for 10–14 days

Table 16.3. Oral desensitization protocol

Penicillin V suspension dose[b]	Amount[a] (units/mL)	mL	Units	Cumulative dose (units)
1	1,000	0.1	100	100
2	1,000	0.2	200	300
3	1,000	0.4	400	700
4	1,000	0.8	800	1,500
5	1,000	1.6	1,600	3,100
6	1,000	3.2	3,200	6,300
7	1,000	6.4	6,400	12,700
8	10,000	1.2	12,000	24,700
9	10,000	2.4	24,000	48,700
10	10,000	4.8	48,000	96,700
11	80,000	1.0	80,000	176,700
12	80,000	2.0	160,000	336,700
13	80,000	4.0	320,000	656,700
14	80,000	8.0	640,000	1,296,700

Observation period: 30 minutes before parenteral administration of penicillin.

[a] Interval between doses: 15 minutes; elapsed time: 3 hours and 45 minutes; and cumulative dose: 1.3 million units.

[b] The specific amount of drug is diluted in approximately 30 mL of water and then administered orally.

Source: Wendel GD Jr, Stark BJ, Jamison RB, et al. Penicillin allergy and desensitization in serious infections during pregnancy. *New Engl J Med* 1985; **312**: 1229–1232.

among men). Risk factors for infection in pregnancy are listed in Table 16.4. Approximately 1.2% of women aged 15–24 test positive during pregnancy. Concomitant chlamydial infection is present in about 40% of pregnant women infected with gonorrhea.

Untreated gonococcal cervicitis is associated with septic spontaneous abortion. Preterm delivery, premature rupture of membranes, chorioamnionitis, and postpartum infection are more common in women with *Neisseria gonorrheae* detected at delivery. Neonatal infections are manifest most commonly as ophthalmia neonatorum, scalp abscess, or disseminated disease.

Table 16.4. Risk factors for gonorrhea infection in pregnancy

Age < 25 years

Unmarried

Previous gonorrheal infection or other sexually transmitted disease

Commercial sex work

New or multiple sex partners

Inconsistent condom use

Drug abuse

Poverty

Diagnosis

Diagnosis of gonococcal infections can be made using culture, nucleic acid hybridization tests, or nucleic acid amplification techniques (NAATs). NAATs have the advantage of utilizing not only endocervical swabs, but also samples collected through less invasive methods such as vaginal swabs and urine. Product inserts from the individual NAAT vendors must be carefully examined, because the specimen types that are FDA-cleared for use vary by test. Vaginal swabs, whether clinician or self-collected, have a comparable sensitivity and specificity, though information specifically from screening among pregnant patients is limited.

All pregnant women at risk for gonorrhea (see Table 16.4) or living in an area of high incidence of gonorrhea should be screened at her first prenatal visit. Uninfected high-risk women should be rescreened in the third trimester.

Treatment

One of the most important problems in gonorrhea treatment has been the emergence of antibiotic-resistant isolates. Resistance to penicillin and tetracycline developed at least 30 years ago and more recently fluoroquinolone resistance has emerged. The Gonococcal Isolate Surveillance Project (GISP) now reports diminished sensitivity of *Neisseria gonorrheae* to azithromycin and to cefixime. Because of these changes and the high rate of coinfection with chlamydia, for effective treatment of gonorrhea infections, two antibiotics are recommended. Ceftriaxone is the most effective cephalosporin for treatment of gonorrhea. The CDC is currently recommending ceftriaxone 250 mg intramuscularly plus azithromycin 1 g orally as the most effective treatment for uncomplicated gonorrhea (Table 16.5). If ceftriaxone is not an option, cefixime 400 mg orally plus azithromycin 1 g orally could be used. The pharmacokinetic parameters of ceftriaxone measured in pregnant patients during the third trimester are similar to those in nonpregnant women. The pharmacokinetic of azithromycin include sustained tissue concentrations, targeted delivery to sites of infection, and lack of significant drug interactions. No alteration in dose is suggested for pregnancy.

Because of emerging antibiotic resistance and the possibility of treatment failure, prompt

Table 16.5. Recommended regimen for gonorrhea during pregnancy

Uncomplicated infection	Ceftriaxone 250 mg IM in a single dose, AND Azithromycin 1 g orally

recognition of cephalosporin-resistant gonorrhea is critical and thus early retesting should be considered. Clinicians caring for pregnant women with gonorrhea infection, particularly in the western United States, might consider having patients return 1 week after treatment for test-of-cure with culture preferably, or with nucleic acid amplification tests (NAATs) at least 3 weeks after therapy. These women should certainly be retested in the third trimester. Screening for other STIs including syphilis, HIV, and *Chlamydia trachomatis* should precede treatment.

Gonococcal bacteremia may lead to petechial or pustular skin lesions, arthralgias, septic arthritis, or tenosynovitis. Pregnant women may account for a disproportionate number of cases of disseminated gonococcal infection in women. Endocarditis rarely complicates pregnancy, but it may be fatal. Because of the rarity of these conditions, consultation with experts in infectious disease should be considered.

Chlamydial infections

Chlamydia is the most commonly reported notifiable disease in the United States with a total of 1,244,180 cases reported to the Centers for Disease Control and Prevention in 2009. Accounting for underreporting, there are an estimated 2.8 million new cases annually. The prevalence of chlamydia in pregnancy varies, depending on population demographics with average rates of approximately 3–7%.

The effect of asymptomatic chlamydial infection on pregnancy outcome remains controversial. The risk of spontaneous abortion does not appear to be increased. However, untreated maternal cervical infection with *Chlamydia trachomatis* increases the risk for preterm delivery, premature rupture of the membranes, and perinatal mortality. There is vertical transmission to 30–50% of infants delivered vaginally to infected women, and *C. trachomatis* is the most common identifiable infectious cause of ophthalmia neonatorum.

Screening asymptomatic pregnant women can detect chlamydial infection and there is some evidence that treatment of chlamydial infection during pregnancy improves maternal and neonatal health outcomes. In several observational studies, treated women had a significantly lower incidence of premature rupture of membranes and low birth weight, as well as a higher infant survival rate, compared to treated patients and patients with negative cultures.

Diagnosis

Diagnosis of chlamydial infections can be made using culture, EIA, nucleic acid hybridization tests, or nucleic acid amplification techniques (NAATs) on endocervical specimens. NAATs are the most sensitive of the tests and are most widely used. Some NAATs are FDA-cleared for use on vaginal swabs (whether clinician or self-collected) and tests have comparable sensitivity and specificity to endocervical specimens. Urine testing using the Aptima Combo 2® Assay (GenProbe Inc. San Diego, CA) has been evaluated specifically in pregnancy and appears equivalent to endocervical sampling.

All pregnant women should be screened for chlamydia at the first prenatal visit. Screening during the first trimester might prevent the adverse effects of chlamydia during pregnancy, but supportive evidence for such screening is lacking. Women aged less than 25 years and those at increased risk (see Table 16.4) should be retested during the third trimester to reduce the risk of maternal postnatal complications and chlamydial infection in the infant.

Treatment

Recommended regimens for treatment of chlamydia infection during pregnancy are listed in Table 16.6. Alternatives include erythromycin base 500 mg orally four times a day for 7 days or 250 mg four times a day for 14 days, or erythromycin ethylsuccinate 800 mg orally four times a day for 7 days or 400 mg orally four times a day for 14 days. Erythromycin is associated with an increased frequency of gastrointestinal side effects

Table 16.6. Recommended regimens for chlamydial infection from the Centers for Disease Control

| Uncomplicated infection | Azithromycin 1 g orally in a single dose |
| | Amoxicillin 500 mg orally TID for 7 days |

and doxycycline and ofloxacin are not used during pregnancy. Erythromycin estolate is contraindicated in pregnancy because of drug-related hepatotoxicity.

Reinfection rates are unfortunately common among women. Counseling messages at the time of treatment should include abstinence from sexual intercourse for 7 days after single-dose therapy or until completion of a 7-day regimen. Additionally, women should also abstain from sexual intercourse until all of their sex partners are treated.

To document chlamydial eradication following treatment, pregnant women should be retested (preferably with NAATs) no sooner than 3 weeks after treatment and again at 3 months. Treating pregnant women usually prevents the transmission of *C. trachomatis* to infants during birth.

Human papillomavirus

Of the more than 100 types of human papillomavirus (HPV), over 40 are found in the genital area. HPV types 16 and 18 are most frequently associated with anogenital and some types of oropharyngeal cancer. Nononcogenic HPV types (e.g. HPV types 6 and 11) are the cause of genital warts and recurrent respiratory papillomatosis. Genital HPV infection is often asymptomatic and self limited. While the exact prevalence of infection is unknown, it is estimated that more than 50% of sexually active persons become infected at least once in their lifetime. Life-time number of sexual partners is strongly associated with HPV infection.

> ★ **TIPS & TRICKS**
>
> It is unclear if Cesarean delivery reduces the risk of transmission of human papillomavirus to the newborn; therefore, Cesarean delivery should not be performed solely to prevent respiratory papillomatosis.

Pregnancy increases the development, growth or reappearance of HPV lesions. Due to higher vascularity and hormonal and immunologic alterations, genital warts frequently increase in number, size, and friability during pregnancy. Lesions can sometimes fill the vagina or cover the perineum and increase the risk of bleeding with vaginal delivery. While HPV types 6 and 11 have been associated with respiratory papillomatosis, pregnant women with genital warts should be informed that the risk for papillomatosis in their infants or children is low.

Diagnosis

Genital warts are commonly diagnosed by visual inspection; however, biopsy can be used to confirm infection. The indications for biopsy are presented in Table 16.7. The use of DNA testing for HPV does not alter clinical management and is not recommended. The application of dilute acetic acid is often used to identify lesions attributed to HPV, but this type of testing has limited specificity for the diagnosis of genital HPV infection and is not recommended. The differential diagnosis includes molluscum contagiosum, micropapillomatosis labialis, intradermal nevus, seborrheic keratoses, and amelanotic melanoma.

Pregnant women should undergo screening with cervical cytology (Papanicolau test) at the same frequency as nonpregnant women, although recommendations for their management differ.

Treatment

The primary reason for treating genital warts is the amelioration of symptoms. Physical methods are the preferred treatment of genital warts during pregnancy, but complete resolution may not occur until after delivery. Podophyllin resin, podofilox 0.5% solution or gel, imiquimod 5% cream, and sinecatechins are not currently recommended for use in pregnancy because of concerns about maternal and fetal safety. For symptomatic women with smaller lesions, trichloroacetic or

Table 16.7. Indications for biopsy of suspected condyloma

Lesions do not respond or worsen during treatment

Lesion is atypical

Patient is immune-compromised

Lesions are pigmented, indurated, bleeding or ulcerated

bichloracetic acid in concentrations of 80–90% are effective and can be used safely in pregnancy. A small amount of the solution can be applied to external lesions using a swab and treatment repeated on a weekly basis. Frequently, extensive lesions spontaneously remit after delivery, and waiting until the puerperium prior to intervention could be appropriate.

If the woman is seen several weeks before delivery, large lesions sometimes can be removed by excision, electrocautery, cryosurgery, or laser ablation. Carbon-dioxide laser has been used during pregnancy to remove large Büschke–Lowenstein tumors under anesthesia. When they are large or diffuse, genital warts can complicate vaginal delivery. If lesions are obstructing the birth canal, or if vaginal delivery may result in excessive bleeding, Cesarean delivery is indicated.

HPV types 6 and 11 can cause respiratory papillomatosis in the infant and child, but the role of maternal–infant transmission is unclear. (It is also unclear if Cesarean delivery reduces the risk of transmission to the newborn; therefore, Cesarean delivery should not be performed solely to prevent respiratory papillomatosis.) No current evidence indicates that the reduction in viral DNA that results from antepartum treatment impacts any risk of peripartum transmission.

The Advisory Committee on Immunization Practices does not recommend HPV vaccination for pregnant women.

Trichomonas infections

The prevalence of trichomoniasis in pregnancy is approximately 7–13%. African American women are more likely to be affected with race-specific prevalence rates that are 2–3 time higher than for Caucasian women. About a third of the cases of trichomoniasis may be asymptomatic. When symptoms are present, after an incubation period ranging from 4 to 28 days, about half of the patients present abundant, foamy, foul-smelling vaginal discharge. Pruritus and/or vulvar irritation, hyperemia of the mucosa with reddish plaques, and urinary symptoms such as dysuria and polyuria may also be present.

Infection with *Trichomonas vaginalis* in pregnancy has been associated with the preterm premature rupture of membranes, preterm delivery, and low birthweight infants. The effect of diagnosis and treatment on these outcomes is controversial. In one large clinical trial, asymptomatic women were screened between 16 and 23 weeks and infected women treated with two 2-g doses of metronidazole 48 hours apart and treated again with the same two-dose regimen between 24 to 29 weeks of gestation. Treatment was associated with an increased risk of spontaneous preterm labor and preterm delivery.

Diagnosis

Vaginal trichomoniasis is commonly diagnosed by a microscopy (wet mount) of vaginal secretions, but this has limited sensitivity (60–70% for wet mount). Point-of-care rapid tests include the OSOM Trichomonas Rapid Test (Genzyme Diagnostics, Cambridge, Massachusetts), an immunochromatographic capillary flow dipstick technology, and the Affirm VP III (Becton Dickenson, San Jose, California) which provide results in less than 1 hour. These rapid tests are highly specific (97%), and have better sensitivity than wet mount (>83%). PCR and TMA (transcription mediated amplification) assays for gonorrhea and chlamydia have been modified to add detection of trichomonas and appear to have comparable sensitivity and specificity to the point-of-care tests. Some large laboratories have added these tests which can be performed on vaginal swabs. Culture remains a highly sensitive and specific test, and can be used in women with suspected trichomoniasis, not confirmed by other methods.

Treatment

There is limited data regarding the comparative efficacy of different treatment regimens in pregnancy. If treatment is undertaken, a 2-g single dose of oral metronidazole has been widely used. It does not appear that any dose adjustment is necessary in pregnancy. Because of the potential increase in preterm birth with treatment, patients should be counseled regarding the potential risks and benefits. Symptomatic patients should be considered for treatment regardless of pregnancy stage. In asymptomatic pregnant women, deferral of therapy until after 37 weeks' gestation is an alternative. Untreated patients should be counseled about the continuing risk of sexual transmission to their partners and the use of condoms.

Chemically related to metronidazole, tinidazole has been used widely outside the United States for treatment of trichomoniasis and is currently licensed for use in this country. A 2-g oral dose of tinidazole has overall clinical efficacy equal to metronidazole (90 to 100%), although tinidazole is considered FDA pregnancy category C and its use in the first trimester is not recommended.

Many studies of metronidazole use in pregnancy have failed to detect an association with teratogenic or mutagenic effects in infants, even when it is used in the first trimester. Therefore, metronidazole is considered safe for use in pregnancy and should be used when indicated. During lactation, breastfeeding should be interrupted during the treatment and 24 hours after the last dose of metronidazole, or 72 hours if prescribing tinidazole.

Bacterial vaginosis

Bacterial vaginosis (BV) is considered a polymicrobial clinical syndrome resulting from an imbalance in the normal vaginal flora, with a decrease in the number of acidophilus lactobacillus, and increased anaerobic organisms (including *Gardnerella vaginalis*). BV is the most common lower genital tract syndrome among women of reproductive age. While BV is the most prevalent cause of vaginal discharge and malodor among women who seek evaluation, many women may be asymptomatic.

BV during pregnancy is associated with adverse pregnancy outcomes, including premature rupture of the membranes, preterm labor, preterm birth, chorioamnionitis, postabortion endometritis, and postpartum endometritis. The role of treatment in reducing adverse pregnancy outcomes is controversial.

Diagnosis

BV can be diagnosed by the use of clinical criteria (i.e. Amsel's Diagnostic Criteria) or by Gram stain which is considered the gold standard laboratory method. Amsel's criteria include: homogeneous, thin, white discharge that smoothly coats the vaginal walls; presence of clue cells on microscopic examination; pH of vaginal fluid >4.5; or a fishy odor of vaginal discharge before or after the addition of 10% KOH (i.e. the whiff test). Three of the four are necessary for a diagnosis of BV. Several other tests have been developed for commercial use. The DNA probe-based test for high concentrations of *G. vaginalis* (Affirm VP III, Becton Dickinson, Sparks, Maryland) has a sensitivity of about 90% compared to Gram stain. The prolineaminopeptidase test card (Pip Activity TestCard, Quidel, San Diego, California) and the OSOM BVBlue test are point-of-care tests providing rapid results with a sensitivity of about 90% compared to Gram stain. Although a card test is available for the detection of elevated pH and trimethylamine, it has low sensitivity and specificity and therefore is not recommended. PCR testing to detect BV-associated organisms is not currently available for use in clinical settings.

The United States Preventive Services Task Force (USPSTF) recently reviewed the utility of BV screening in pregnancy and found no evidence to support screening or treating low-risk pregnant women asymptomatic for BV. Similarly, they found no benefit to screening for, and treating, BV in the general population of pregnant women who are asymptomatic for BV. Studies of screening and treating women at high risk for preterm delivery are conflicting regarding benefits and harms. Studies in high-risk populations have shown reductions in preterm birth, no effect, and, in one case, increased rates of preterm birth.

Treatment

All symptomatic pregnant women should be tested and treated. Recommended regimens for treatment are listed in Table 16.8. Meta-analyses have demonstrated no increase in teratogenic or mutagenic effect associated with metronidazole use during pregnancy. Intravaginal clindamycin

Table 16.8. Treatment regimens for bacterial vaginosis recommended by Centers for Disease Control

Metronidazole 500 mg orally twice a day for 7 days
Metronidazole 250 mg orally three times a day for 7 days
Clindamycin 300 mg orally twice a day for 7 days

is not recommended during pregnancy, particularly after 20 weeks. In several studies, intravaginal clindamycin cream administered at 16–32 weeks' gestation was associated with an increase in low birth weight and neonatal infections and no reduction in rates of preterm birth. Treatment of sex partners is not recommended.

Because of the potential risk for post-operative infectious complications associated with BV, some providers screen and treat women with BV in addition to providing routine antimicrobial prophylaxis before abortions. However, more information is needed before recommending treatment of asymptomatic BV before these procedures, particularly Cesarean delivery.

Summary

Women and children often bear a disproportionate burden from sexually transmitted infections. STIs are strongly related to preterm delivery, low birth weight, and increased morbidity and mortality. Physicians and other healthcare providers play an essential role in preventing and treating STDs. Attention to the specific needs of pregnant women is critical to reduce the risks of adverse outcomes.

Bibliography

American College of Obstetricians Gynecologists. Management of herpes in pregnancy. *Obstet Gynecol* 2007; **109**: 1489–1498.

Centers for Disease Control and Prevention (CDC). Seroprevalence of herpes simplex virus type 2 among persons aged 14–49 years – United States, 2005–2008. *MMWR*. 2010; **59**(15): 456–459.

Centers for Disease Control and Prevention. Cephalosporin sensitivity among *Neisseria gonorrhoeae* isolates in the United States, 2000–2010. *MMWR* 2011; **60**(26): 873–877.

Centers for Disease Control and Prevention. Sexually Transmitted Diseases Treatment Guidelines, 2010. *MMWR* 2010; **59** (No. RR-12): 1–75.

Centers for Disease Control and Prevention. *Sexually Transmitted Disease Surveillance 2009.* U.S. Department of Health and Human Services: Atlanta, 2010.

Cohen I, Veille JC, Calkins BM. Improved pregnancy outcome following successful treatment of chlamydial infection. *J Am Med Assoc* 1990: **263;** 3160–3163.

Davison JM, Hytten FE. The effect of pregnancy on the renal handling of glucose. *Br J Obstet Gynaecol* 1975; **82**: 374–381.

Donders G. Diagnosis and management of bacterial vaginosis and other types of abnormal vaginal bacterial flora: a review. *Obstet Gynecol Surv.* 2010; **65**(7): 462–473.

Garland SM, Steben M, Sings HL, et al. Natural history of genital warts: analysis of the placebo arm of 2 randomized phase III trials of a quadrivalent human papillomavirus (types 6, 11, 16, and 18) vaccine. *J Infect Dis* 2009; **199**: 805–814.

Garozzo G, Nuciforo G, Rocchi CM, et al. Büschke-Lowenstein tumour in pregnancy. *Eur J Obstet Gynecol Reprod Biol.* 2003; **111**(1): 88–90.

Gaydos CA, Cartwright CP, Colaninno P, et al. Performance of the Abbott RealTime CT/NG for detection of Chlamydia trachomatis and Neisseria gonorrhoeae. *J Clin Microbiol.* 2010; **48**(9): 3236–43.

Hollier LM, Wendel GD. Third trimester antiviral prophylaxis for preventing maternal genital herpes simplex virus (HSV) recurrences and neonatal infection. *Cochrane Database Syst Rev.* 2008; **1**: CD004946.

Hosenfeld CB, Workowski KA, Berman S, et al. Repeat infection with Chlamydia and gonorrhea among females: a systematic review of the literature. *Sex Transm Dis.* 2009; **36**(8): 478–489.

Klebanoff MA, Carey JC, Hauth JC, et al. Failure of metronidazole to prevent preterm delivery among pregnant women with asymptomatic *Trichomonas vaginalis* infection. *New Engl J Med* 2001; **345**: 487–493.

McLennon CE, Thouin LG. Blood volume in pregnancy. *Am J Obstet Gynecol* 1948; **55**: 1189.

Nygren P, Fu R, Freeman M, Bougatsos C, Guise JM. Screening and Treatment for Bacterial Vaginosis in Pregnancy: Systematic Review to Update the 2001 U.S. Preventive Services Task Force Recommendation. Rockville (MD): Agency for Healthcare Research and Quality (US); 2008 Jan. Report No.: 08-05106-EF-1.

Ratanajamit C, Vinther Skriver M, Jepsen P, Chongsuvivatwong V, Olsen J, Sorensen HT. Adverse pregnancy outcome in women exposed to acyclovir during pregnancy: a population-based observational study. *Scand J Infect Dis* 2003; **35**: 255–259.

Roberts CM, Pfister JR, Spear SJ. Increasing proportion of herpes simplex virus type 1 as a cause of genital herpes infection in college students. *Sex Transm Dis* 2003; **30**: 797–800.

Roberts SW, Sheffield JS, McIntire DD, Alexander JM. Urine screening for Chlamydia trachomatis during pregnancy. *Obstet Gynecol* 2011; **117**(4): 883–885.

Silverberg MJ, Thorsen P, Lindeberg H, et al. Condyloma in pregnancy is strongly predictive of juvenile-onset recurrent respiratory papillomatosis. *Obstet Gynecol.* 2003; **101**(4): 645–652.

Wendel GD, Jr, Stark BJ, Jamison RB, et al. Penicillin allergy and desensitization in serious infections during pregnancy. *New Engl J Med* 1985; **312**: 1229–1232.

Prevention of Sexually Transmitted Diseases

Michelle H. Moniz and Richard H. Beigi

Department of Obstetrics, Gynecology & Reproductive Sciences,
Division of Reproductive Infectious Diseases, Magee-Womens Hospital of the
University of Pittsburgh Medical Center, Pittsburgh, PA, USA

Background

The term "sexually transmitted diseases" (STDs) encompasses a diverse variety of pathogens (including bacteria, viruses, and parasites) that share a common mode of transmission: sexual behaviors between human beings (see Science Revisited). As a group, sexually transmitted diseases constitute a major public health issue. These diseases are prevalent and are associated with harmful, sometimes irreversible, complications that engender tremendous health and economic consequences. Although STDs are often preventable with behavioral modifications, they are largely under-recognized by patients and healthcare providers.

> ### ⚘ SCIENCE REVISITED
>
> Sexually transmitted diseases are caused by bacteria, viruses, protozoa, fungi, and parasites. This diverse group of etiologic agents has in common their vector of transmission from one person to another: sexual contact. Some of these agents include:
>
> - **Bacteria:** *Neisseria gonorrhea* (gonorrhea), *Chlamydia trachomatis* (chlamydia), *Treponema pallidum* (syphilis), *Hemophilus ducreyi* (chancroid), *Klebsiella granulomatis* (granuloma inguinale)
> - **Viruses:** Human immunodeficiency virus (HIV/AIDS), herpes simplex virus type 1 and type 2 (genital herpes), human papillomavirus (genital warts, cervical dysplasia, and cancer), hepatitis B virus (hepatitis), molluscum contagiosum virus
> - **Parasites:** *Trichomonas vaginalis* (trichomoniasis), pediculus humanus (lice), sarcoptes scabei (scabies)

Prevention is a key component in the control of sexually transmitted diseases, particularly those that are incurable, such as HIV and genital herpes. Because STDs are transmitted by sexual contact between human beings, any viable STD prevention effort must account for the complex network of factors that influence sexual risk-taking behaviors. Additionally, biologic factors – for example, the asymptomatic nature of many sexually transmitted diseases and the often lengthy latency between acquisition and clinical symptoms – should be considered in order to maximize the efficacy of preventive efforts.

Until recently, prevention was an understudied facet of STD research and control programs. Those prevention efforts that did exist were often linked to a moral agenda that propagated fear-based messages about the consequences of depraved behavior. Such efforts frequently neglected consideration of structural factors influencing sexual behaviors (i.e. work requirements engendering spousal separation, barriers to economic independence for women, population displacement, etc.). Newer approaches incorporate consideration of the socio-behavioral factors that influence the spread of STDs, particularly among vulnerable populations. It should also be noted that existing techniques for STD prevention are primarily biomedical in nature and there exists relatively little systemic data on behavioral science approaches to behavioral change for STD prevention.

Physicians play an integral role in preventing disease transmitted through sexual activity. Obstetrician gynecologists (Ob/Gyns) in particular have a unique opportunity to provide sexual education to their patients as they are experienced at taking a detailed sexual history, assessing for STD risk factors, and counseling patients about STDs and safer sexual behaviors. Additionally, they may establish lasting relationships with patients through regular annual examinations and prenatal care visits, and may be in a unique and privileged position to advise and counsel patients about safe sexual decision-making.

Based on the data available, the Centers for Disease Control and Prevention (CDC), the US Preventive Services Task Force, the American Congress of Obstetricians and Gynecologists, and other professional organizations have put forth recommendations to assist healthcare providers in promoting clinical prevention of STDs. This chapter will provide a brief overview of STD prevention techniques for use in the office-based counseling of individual patients.

Conceptualizing prevention

In order to foster an understanding of the field of STD prevention, it is necessary to define a few terms. Applied to STDs, *prevention* refers to any action taken to mitigate an anticipated untoward outcome from the sexually transmitted pathogens. STD prevention efforts can be divided into primary and secondary interventions. *Primary prevention* refers to deterrence of the first occurrence of the disease. These are often interventions to change the sexual behaviors that put a person at risk for infection in order to prevent the initial acquisition of the disease. *Secondary prevention* efforts seek to avert or mitigate complications or recurrence of the disease among those already infected and to reduce ongoing transmission.

The classification of STD prevention efforts can also be based on their target: individuals, groups, or populations. Those targeting individuals likely will be most relevant to the Ob/Gyn's practice. The advantages of individual-level interventions include the ability to tailor them to the particular needs of a given patient. Weaknesses include the time and labor (and ensuing cost) involved and the difficulty of identifying those patients who would benefit most from the intervention.

The CDC identifies five major strategies that can be implemented in the office for the prevention and control of STDs:

1. Education and counseling of at-risk patients.
2. Identification of infected patients unlikely to receive treatment (asymptomatic or unlikely to seek healthcare services).
3. Effective diagnosis, treatment and counseling of infected persons.
4. Effective diagnosis, treatment and counseling of sex partners of infected persons.
5. Pre-exposure vaccination of individuals at risk for STDs.

When considering STD prevention for an individual patient, the healthcare provider should consider the individual's risk factors for disease acquisition, possibility of transmission and likelihood of progression to clinically significant disease. Some variables that might affect an individual's risk include: age, type of partnership (heterosexual, homosexual or bisexual), specific clinical circumstances, gender power dynamics within the relationship, local disease prevalence, cultural norms, and healthcare-seeking behavior.

Std prevention counseling

> **★ TIPS & TRICKS 1**
>
> Use the 5 Ps recommended by the CDC to help obtain a thorough sexual history.
>
> **The 5 Ps**
>
> 1. Partners: Men, women or both? Lifetime partners? Current partners? Monogamy?
> 2. Prevention of Pregnancy: What are you doing to prevent pregnancy?
> 3. Protection from STDs: How do you protect yourself against STDs?
> 4. Practices: Vaginal, anal, oral sex? Condoms?
> 5. Past History of STDs (in patient or patient's partners)
>
> *Adapted from:* Centers for Disease Control and Prevention. *Sexually Transmitted Diseases Treatment Guidelines, 2010*

The CDC recommends the following: "as part of the clinical interview, healthcare providers should routinely and regularly obtain sexual histories from their patients and address management of risk reduction." A thorough sexual history can help to identify individual sexual behaviors that contribute to risk for STDs. The CDC has defined the "5 Ps" approach as an interactive counseling technique to assess a patient's **Part**ners, **P**revention of pregnancy, **P**rotection from STDs, **P**ractices, and **P**ast history of STDs.

Patients and physicians may both have difficulty conversing candidly about sexual issues. The use of open-ended questions and understandable, normalizing language can help providers to obtain an accurate sexual history (see Tips & Tricks 2).

> **★ TIPS & TRICKS 2**
>
> The following techniques may enhance your interviewing skills:
>
> 1. Use open-ended questions: "What are you doing to prevent STDs? Tell me about your experience with condoms. Tell me about any new sexual partners you've had since we last met."
> 2. Use understandable language: "Have you ever had a sore/bump/rash on your vagina?"

> 3. Use normalizing language: "Some of my patients have difficulty using a condom with every single act of sex. How do you do with this?"

Obtaining a detailed sexual history is only the first part of STD prevention counseling. After identifying an individual patient's risk factors for STDs, providers should deliver prevention messages and encourage risk-reduction behavioral changes. Risk-reduction messages should be relevant to the individual patient and should incorporate a discussion of specific actions that can reduce the risk of STD acquisition/transmission (abstinence, condom use, vaccination, etc.).

A provider's approach to sexual interviewing and counseling should communicate respect, empathy, and a nonjudgmental attitude. Providers should seek to tailor the preventive message to the individual's language, developmental level, culture, sex, sexual orientation and behaviors, and age. Most risk behaviors are not distributed randomly in populations, but rather tend to cluster. Known vulnerable populations include: adolescents, female sex workers and their clients, homosexual and bisexual persons, illegal drug users, and migrant populations (see Tips & Tricks 3). Counseling efforts should be heightened when treating these patients.

> **★ TIPS & TRICKS 3**
>
> Prevention counseling may be particularly rewarding in individuals from high-risk populations, including:
>
> - adolescents
> - female sex workers and their clients
> - homosexual and bisexual persons
> - individuals using illegal drugs
> - refugee and immigrant populations.

Prevention methods

Office-based counseling for STD prevention (see Tips & Tricks 4) should incorporate a brief review of the available methods of preventing STD acquisition and spread.

Abstinence and reduction in number of sex partners

The most effective way of preventing STD acquisition is the avoidance of oral, vaginal, and anal sex, which all involve contact between body parts or fluids that facilitate pathogenic transmission. Providers can counsel patients that a delay of sexual initiation and a reduction in the total number of lifetime partners may reduce an individual's risk of acquiring a STD.

For currently abstinent patients planning on initiating sexual activity, providers can recommend that both partners undergo STD screening prior to the initiation of sexual contact, or prior to resuming contact if one person has had sexual relations with another individual. Patients should be educated about the limitations of STD screening, including the fact that many STDs are not detectable immediately after exposure and that some STDs, particularly latent viruses like HSV, may be difficult to detect with current screening methods. Abstinence is also important for individuals undergoing treatment for a STD; it is critical to counsel patients about the importance of abstinence until completion of medical therapy to avoid reinfection with a STD (see Tips & Tricks 5).

Abstinence will not be a feasible, sustainable strategy for many, if not most patients, so providers can consider mentioning the methods listed below, even with patients who currently plan to abstain from sexual activity.

Immunization against STDs

Pre-exposure vaccination is a highly effective method of preventing STD transmission. At present, vaccines are available for HPV and hepatitis A and B. Two commercially available HPV vaccines are: the quadrivalent Gardasil® and the bivalent Cervarix®. Gardasil® prevents acquisition of HPV types 16, 18, 6, and 11, the viral types are responsible for most cervical dysplasia and genital warts. The vaccine is recommended for females and males age 9–26 to prevent HPV infection and is ideally given before the first sexual contact. The HPV vaccines will be discussed in detail elsewhere in this book. Hepatitis A is frequently a self-limited liver disease caused by the hepatitis A virus. The route of transmission is primarily fecal–oral. Hepatitis B tends to cause a more serious disease with the potential for chronic illness and long-term complications. Hepatitis B is transmitted via percutaneous (skin puncture) or mucosal contact. Vaccination is the most effective way to prevent infection with either hepatitis virus. The CDC recommends hepatitis B vaccination for all uninfected, unvaccinated individuals presenting for STD screening or treatment. Both the hepatitis A and B vaccines are recommended by the CDC for all men who have sex with men and for patients who use intravenous drugs. There is a newly available combined hepatitis A/hepatitis B vaccine, Twinrix®, that providers can consider offering to appropriate patients.

Condoms

Condoms serve as an impermeable barrier to STD pathogens. Even when used correctly, the male condom will provide differential levels of protection based on the method of pathogenic transmission. Some STDs, like HIV, trichomoniasis, gonorrhea, and chlamydia, are transmitted when infected vaginal or urethral secretions contact a mucosal surface, like the cervix, vagina, or male urethra. Other STDs, including HPV and the genital ulcerative diseases like herpes and syphilis, are transmitted via contact with infected skin or mucosa. Greater protection is afforded against diseases transmitted in genital secretions, with a lesser degree of protection against the genital ulcerative diseases, which can transmit via skin/mucosa not covered by a condom.

Condom effectiveness has been extensively examined in multiple epidemiologic studies of couples serodiscordant for HIV. Numerous well-designed studies suggest that consistent, correct condom use is highly effective for preventing HIV transmission. Condoms also provide a high degree of protection against other STDs, like gonorrhea, chlamydia, and trichomoniasis. There also exists data to suggest that latex condoms reduce the risk of transmission of the genital ulcerative diseases, but only when the active lesions are in areas covered by the condom. Similarly, condoms may reduce the risk of HPV infection when the condom covers infected areas.

Providers should carefully counsel patients about the importance of the consistent and correct use of condoms to maximize their effectiveness. Condom failure to prevent STD transmission usually results from improper use and not from product failure (see Tips & Tricks 6). Patients should be clearly instructed to use a new condom with every act of oral, vaginal, and anal sex and to use it throughout the sex act.

★ TIPS & TRICKS 6

Counsel patients about the four major mistakes that put them at risk for condom failure.

1. Failure to use condoms with every act of genital contact: use a condom every time.
2. Failure to use throughout intercourse.
3. Condom breakage and slippage: (a) if suspected, the sex act should stop, the condom should be removed, and a new condom should be applied; (b) consider using a back-up method for pregnancy prevention.
4. Improper lubricant use: oil-based lubricants can compromise the structural integrity of latex and should not be used.

Two types of male condom made from non-latex materials are available. The first type is synthetic and can be used by persons with latex allergies. Synthetic nonlatex male condoms have higher breakage rates than latex condoms, but the pregnancy rates among women whose partners use synthetic or latex condoms are the same. The second type of nonlatex condom is the natural membrane condom, typically made from lamb intestines. These condoms function as a barrier to sperm, but are permeable to viral particles. Thus, natural membrane condoms are not recommended for STD prevention.

The male latex condom has been studied in conjunction with spermicides. Condoms lubricated with spermicides appear to be no more effective in preventing STD transmission than other lubricated condoms. Furthermore, frequent spermicide use can predispose to erosion of the genital mucosa, increasing susceptibility to HIV acquisition. Spermicide-coated condoms are more expensive, have a shorter shelf-life, and have been associated with urinary tract infections in women. For all of these reasons, condoms lubricated with spermicide are not recommended for STD prevention.

The female condom (Reality) has been shown to be an effective barrier to sexually transmitted pathogens, including such viruses as HIV. They are generally more expensive than male condoms, but are available as an alternative barrier method for interested patients.

The promotion of condoms in some communities is controversial, based on a belief that increased availability of condoms will increase sexual activity. It should be remembered that multiple studies suggest that the endorsement and availability of condoms does not increase the frequency of sexual behavior. Office-based counseling should indisputably communicate the scientific evidence for condom effectiveness in STD prevention.

Pre-exposure prophylaxis

Ongoing research has suggested that both oral and vaginal use of antiretroviral drugs can prevent new HIV infections in both women and men. While promising, larger studies will determine the efficacy of these approaches, and whether widespread availability is warranted.

Partner management

When a patient is diagnosed with a STD, it is important for the healthcare provider to promote treatment of infected partners and to abort further disease transmission. It is important to counsel patients diagnosed with a STD to disclose this to their partners and urge them to seek testing and treatment. Partner treatment has been shown to reduce rates of reinfection in the index patient. Patient-delivered partner therapy has been shown to reduce recurrence rates in the index patient. Expedited partner therapy is prohibited, or the topic of ongoing legislation, in some states, so providers should verify local legalities and availability of this strategy for STD prevention.

Special populations

Pregnant women

All pregnant women are at risk for having acquired STDs as STDs can have particularly untoward effects on pregnancy and neonatal outcomes. Pregnancy represents a time of frequent healthcare visits and heightened patient motivation to improve health; as such, pregnancy might be a particularly opportune time to deliver STD screening and counseling. The CDC makes the following recommendations regarding STD screening in pregnant women:

1. *HIV:* Screen all pregnant women at their initial prenatal visit, or as early as possible, via opt-out screening. Retest in the third trimester for high-risk women (those who use illicit drugs, have had STDs during pregnancy, have multiple sex partners during pregnancy, live in areas with a high prevalence of HIV, or have HIV-infected partners). Send rapid HIV screening on any woman in labor with an undocumented HIV status unless she declines.
2. *Syphilis:* Screen all pregnant women at their initial prenatal visit, or as early as possible. Repeat testing in high-risk women (live in areas of high syphilis morbidity) or those who were previously untested early in the third trimester (at approximately 28 weeks' gestation) and at delivery.
3. *Hepatitis* B: Screen all pregnant women at their initial prenatal visit, or as early as possible. Retest at time of delivery in those with clinical hepatitis or high-risk women (more than one sex partner in the past 6 months, evaluations/treatment for STD during pregnancy, intravenous drug use, sex partner positive for HBsAg).
4. *Gonorrhea:* Screen all pregnant women at their initial prenatal visit, or as early as possible. Repeat testing in the third trimester for high-risk women (age <25, prior gonorrhea infection, other STDs, new/multiple sex partners, commercial sex work, drug use).
5. *Chlamydia:* Screen all pregnant women at their initial prenatal visit, or as early as possible. Repeat testing in the third trimester for high-risk women (age <25, new sex partner).
6. Routine screening is NOT recommended for BV, trichomonas, and HSV-2. Women presenting with symptoms concerning for these diseases should be evaluated and treated as indicated.

Adolescents

In the United States, reported prevalence rates of many STDs are highest among adolescents. The majority of adolescents (70% of adolescent females and 65% of adolescent males – see Tips & Tricks 7) have had penile-vaginal sex by age 19. Sexual initiation in adolescents is accompanied by a considerable risk of STDs and pregnancy. Ob/Gyns are uniquely positioned to mitigate these risks by educating young patients about safe sexual decision-making. Providers should ask frequently about sexual behaviors and anticipate frequent changes in sexual behaviors over time in this population.

> ☆ **TIPS & TRICKS 7**
>
> 70% of adolescent females and 65% of adolescent males have had sex by age 19. Ask frequently about sexual behaviors and anticipate changes over time. Provide skills and education promoting safe sexual decision-making even for those currently refraining.

STD prevention in adolescents poses unique challenges. There exist powerful developmental influences (biological, psychological, and social) on adolescent sexual behavior. Cognitive immaturity, despite advancing physical development, may preclude understanding and implementation of risk-reduction strategies. Adolescents have fewer cumulative life experiences and may not have the skills to navigate difficult conversations and negotiate safer-sex behaviors with their partners. Additionally, adolescents may have different definitions of "sex" and "abstinence" than do most adults. Adolescents may not view sex and abstinence as mutually exclusive (see Tips & Tricks 8). Adolescents often do not consider oral or anal genital contact as "sex," despite the fact that these behaviors put them at risk for STDs. Adolescents who state they are "abstinent," and who deny engaging in penile-vaginal sex, have often engaged in noncoital sexual behaviors that increase their risk of acquiring a STD.

☆ TIPS & TRICKS 8

Remember that adolescents tend to conceptualize abstinence differently than adults, with significant variation by gender, age, and sexual experience. They may not view abstinence and sex as mutually exclusive.

Clinical data on counseling adolescents about STD and pregnancy prevention in the office setting are sparse, with studies heterogeneous in design and often poor in quality. Little is definitively know about appropriate content, length, delivery format, and theoretical basis. Existing data suggest that STD risk assessment and gender-specific, culturally-tailored, clinic-based educational interventions can enhance STD-preventive behaviors and skills in adolescents. A brief, office-based discussion appears to be as effective as more enhanced educational efforts at preventing STDs in adolescents. Skills-based counseling is probably more effective that didactic counseling. Some tips for office-based counseling of adolescents (based primarily on expert opinion) are presented in Tips & Tricks 9.

☆ TIPS & TRICKS 9

Office-based STD prevention counseling of the adolescent patient

1. Use concrete language and refer to specific behaviors.
   - (a) *Clarify terminology:*
     - i. "What do you consider to be sex?"
     - ii. Use the phrase "not having sex" instead of abstinence.
   - (b) *Use open-ended questions:*
     - i. "What have you decided about how far to go sexually?"
     - ii. "Have you ever thought about having sex with anyone?
     - iii. "What do you do to protect yourself from STDs?"
   - (c) *Normalize the behaviors you're discussing:*
     - i. "Do any of your friends use condoms?"
     - ii. "Do you know anyone with an STD?"
     - iii. "Have any of your relationships involved sexual activity?"
   - (d) *Give choices for the questions you ask:*
     - i. "Using condoms can be difficult. For you, is it challenging because they're expensive, it's hard to remember to use them, they aren't always available, you don't like using them, or some other reason I haven't thought of?"
     - ii. "Do you consider yourself to be straight, gay or lesbian, bisexual, something else, or you're not sure?"
2. Replace a knowledge-based approach with an interactive, skill-building, problem-solving approach:
     - i. "If he says ...., what would you say?"
     - ii. "Some of my adolescent patients feel that .... What would you say to them?")
3. Ask permission: "Would it be ok if I told you about ...."

The CDC recommend that providers inquire about sexual behaviors, assess STD risks, and offer risk-reduction counseling and STD screening to adolescents. The following recommendations for STD screening and primary prevention can be considered:

1. Annual screening for gonorrhea and chlamydia for all sexually active females at $</=$25 years.
2. Cervical cancer screening via Pap smear beginning at age 21.
3. HPV vaccination at age 9–11 years (with catch up vaccination up to age 26).
4. Hepatitis A and B vaccination for all adolescents who have not already received the series.
5. Compulsory counseling about STD transmission and complications for all adolescents.

Screening can be discussed with all adolescents and encouraged for those who are sexually active.

Women who have sex with women

Women who have sex with women (WSW) are at risk of acquiring STDs from current or prior partners, both male and female. Therefore, counseling and screening recommendations are no different among WSW than among women who have sex only with men.

Clinical data on STD prevalence and risk behaviors in this population is limited, with most studies involving direct measurement of common STDs in small patient populations or surveys to collect self-reported data on sexual behaviors. There is little, if any, data from national, state or local STD-reporting systems. Practices involving infected cervicovaginal secretions and contact between oral, vaginal, and anal surfaces provide a biologically plausible mechanism for STD transmission. Indeed, the medical literature reports on the transmission of genotype-concordant HIV, metronidazole-resistant trichomoniasis, and genital warts between WSW. Transmission of chlamydia, HSV, and syphilis has also been documented, and screening guidelines for these STDs are no different for WSW than for women with solely heterosexual behaviors. It is known that transmission of HPV is observed via skin-to-skin or mucosal contact, which can readily occur in the context of lesbian sex. Furthermore, many self-identified WSW report having had sex with a man at some point and acknowledge the possibility of future such encounters.

Thus, all women should be offered routine cervical cancer screening, regardless of their sexual identity, preferences, or practices.

In addition to screening for STDs, routine counseling on sexual risk-reduction strategies is indicated in WSW, and counseling should emphasize the plausibility of STD transfer between female partners. It may be helpful to discuss the cleaning of shared sex objects between uses to reduce the chances of transfer of vaginal secretions/flora between partners. Providers can discuss barriers methods, including dental dams for oral–vaginal and oral–anal sex and condoms for penetrative sex acts. Hand-hygiene in association with penetrative sex should also be reviewed. Providers should also note that many WSW abstain from or underutilize healthcare services because of perceived or real homophobia. Some data suggests that WSW are less likely to receive gynecologic services and use contraceptives. Providers should strive to deliver respectful, knowledgeable care to this sometimes marginalized population.

Conclusions

Healthcare providers make a vital contribution to STD prevention by providing individualized, nonjudgmental risk-reduction counseling to patients in the office-based setting. STD prevention methods that might be helpful for individual patients include: abstinence, reduction in number of sexual partners, immunization against STDs, condom use, pre-exposure prophylaxis, and partner management. Some populations, including pregnant women, adolescents, and women who have sex with women, may require special consideration of their unique screening and counseling needs. Resources for the provider seeking to learn more about STD prevention can be found on the CDC's website (http://www.cdc.gov/STD/training/courses.htm).

Bibliography

Centers for Disease Control and Prevention. Sexually Transmitted Diseases Treatment Guidelines, 2010. *MMWR* 2010; **59**(No. RR-12): 1–110.

Centers for Disease Control and Prevention. *Condoms and STDs: Fact Sheet for Public Health Personnel.* Available at http://www.cdc.gov/

condomeffectiveness/latex.htm (accessed 6/9/11).

Centers for Disease Control and Prevention. *Expedited Partner Therapy in the Management of Sexually Transmitted Diseases*. US Department of Health and Human Services: Atlanta, GA, 2006.

Centers for Disease Control and Prevention. *STDs and Pregnancy Fact Sheet*. Available at http://www.cdc.gov/std/pregnancy/STDFact-Pregnancy.htm (accessed 6/9/11).

King Holmes, et al. (eds.). *Sexually Transmitted Diseases*. McGraw-Hill Companies, Inc., 2008.

Marrazzo JM, et al. Sexual practices, risk perception, and knowledge of sexually transmitted disease risk among lesbian and bisexual women. *Persp Sex Reprod Health* 2005; **37**(1): 6–12.

Marrazzo JM. Barriers to infectious disease care among lesbians. *Emerg Infect Dis* 2004; **10**(11): 1974–1978.

Monasterio E, et al. Adolescent sexual health. *Curr Prob Pediat Adoles Health Care* 2007; **37** (8): 302–325.

Pedlow CT, Carey MP. Developmentally appropriate sexual risk reduction interventions for adolescents: rationale. Review of interventions, and recommendations for research and practice. *Ann Behav Med* 2004; **27**: 172–184.

Piper JM. Prevention of sexually transmitted infections in women. *Infect Dis Clin North Am*. 2008 Dec; **22**(4): 619–635, v–vi.

Index

Note: page numbers in *italics* refer to figures, those in **bold** refer to tables and boxes

Sexually Transmitted Diseases, First Edition. Edited by Richard H. Beigi.
© 2012 John Wiley & Sons, Ltd. Published 2012 by John Wiley & Sons, Ltd.

Sexually Transmitted Diseases

This book is dedicated to all of my excellent mentors and to my family for their ongoing support.